Transgender Children and Young People

Transgender Children and Young People:

Born in Your Own Body

Edited by

Heather Brunskell-Evans
and Michele Moore

Cambridge
Scholars
Publishing

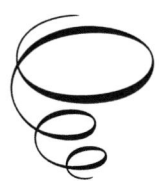

Transgender Children and Young People: Born in Your Own Body

Edited by Heather Brunskell-Evans and Michele Moore

This book first published 2018

Cambridge Scholars Publishing

Lady Stephenson Library, Newcastle upon Tyne, NE6 2PA, UK

British Library Cataloguing in Publication Data
A catalogue record for this book is available from the British Library

Copyright © 2018 by Heather Brunskell-Evans, Michele Moore
and contributors

All rights for this book reserved. No part of this book may be reproduced, stored in a retrieval system, or transmitted, in any form or by any means, electronic, mechanical, photocopying, recording or otherwise, without the prior permission of the copyright owner.

ISBN (10): 1-5275-0398-4
ISBN (13): 978-1-5275-0398-4

This book is dedicated to children living with gender confusion.

Contents

Contributors ix

Chapter One 1
The Fabrication of 'The Transgender Child'
Heather Brunskell Evans and Michele Moore

Chapter Two 16
The Transgender Experiment on Children
Stephanie Davies-Arai

Chapter Three 41
Gendered Mis-Intelligence: The Fabrication of 'The Transgender Child'
Heather Brunskell-Evans

Chapter Four 64
'I'm Not A Hideously Bigoted Parent Who Doesn't 'Get' It'
GenderCriticalDad

Chapter Five 87
'Trans' Kids: LGB Adults Come Out
Josephine Bartosch

Chapter Six 107
The Language of the Psyche: Symptoms as Symbols
Lisa Marchiano

Chapter Seven 123
The Body Factory: Twentieth Century Stories of Sex Change
Susan Matthews

Chapter Eight 139
A Full Life Uninterrupted by Transition
Miranda Yardley

Chapter Nine 166
Unheard Voices of Detransitioners
Carey Maria Catt Callahan

Chapter Ten 181
The View from the Consulting Room
Robert Withers

Chapter Eleven 201
Trans Utopias: Transhumanism, Transfeminism and Manufacturing the Self
Jen Izaakson

Chapter Twelve 218
Standing Up for Girls and Boys
Michele Moore

Contributors

Josephine Bartosch
Jo Bartosch founded the group Chelt Fems, a network of feminist activists, academics and professionals. She then became co-director of 'Critical Sisters' which offers a platform for marginal feminist opinion with particular emphasis on unravelling the twin man-made beliefs of gender and religion. She has authored several reports exploring the links between violence against women and commercial sexual entertainment. She is a frequently commissioned journalist, recently publishing the powerful article *What about the children who said they were transgender – and then changed their minds?* Independent (2017)

Heather Brunskell-Evans
Heather is a social theorist and philosopher, Senior Research Fellow at King's College, London, UK. She has a longstanding interest in the work of Michel Foucault and in feminist philosophy and politics of the body. She is a Trustee of FiLia and Director of its *Stop Violence against Women and Girls* section. Heather has published extensively including most recently: *The Sexualized Body and the Medical Authority of Pornography*, Cambridge Scholars (2016). You can follow her on Twitter @brunskellevans and read more of her writing at www.heather-brunskell-evans.co.uk

Carey Maria Catt Callahan
Carey Maria Catt Callahan is a detransitioned woman, family therapy trainee, and writer living in Cleveland, Ohio, USA. Through her videos, writing, and public speaking she advocates for awareness and greater clinical support for detransitioned people. She wants people to do well. You can follow her on Twitter @catt_bear and engage with her writing and videos https://careycallahan.com

Stephanie Davies-Arai
Stephanie Davies-Arai is a communication skills trainer who has worked with parents and teachers for over 18 years. She was one of the founders of a successful Small School in Lewes UK and is author of the blog and the book *Communicating with Kids*. She was a prominent member of the successful No More Page 3 campaign and is an experienced speaker on

parenting, feminism and 'transgender' kids. She founded and runs the website *Transgender Trend* www.transgendertrend.com an information and research-based resource for parents and everyone concerned about the current trend to 'transition' children you can follow on Twitter @Transgendertrd. Follow Stephanie on Twitter @cwknews and www.stephaniedaviesarai.com

GenderCriticalDad
I'm a middle of the road middle aged dad trying to keep his daughter safe. Lefty liberal newspaper reader, organic eggs and chicken, equal shares sort of dad. I earn my living making machines doing stuff for people, fixing their machines when they don't work. My daughter is being damaged by transgender dogma. I hate what it's doing to her, but I love her. As I cannot critique transgender dogma without harming her I write anonymously. I write a blog *http://gendercriticaldad.blogspot.co.uk* which gained far more attention than I ever imagined possible. It grew in to *http://gendercriticaldad.blogspot.co.uk/2017/* which has details of a support board for parents of gender dysphoric children and young adults I helped set up with https://4thwavenow.com. I readily admit to shamelessly stealing ideas from Gender Critical Radical Feminism. You can follow me on Twitter @dad_gc

Jen Izaakson
Jen Izaakson is a PhD student in the UK at Kingston University's Centre for Research in Modern European Philosophy (CRMEP), researching gender and Freud. Specifically this research focuses on the way in which a Freudian critique of Queer theory can locate the theoretical limits of Queer analysis and how Freud's theory of primary femininity and universal bisexuality can actually tell us more about what is termed 'queer affect'. She recently published her views on sexual assault *The PWR BTTM debacle demonstrates why queer politics don't protect women,* Feminist Current (2017). You can find Jen on Twitter at @isacsohn

Lisa Marchiano
Lisa Marchiano is a licensed clinical social worker and certified Jungian analyst in private practice in Philadelphia, Pennsylvania, USA. She received her MSW from New York University and completed analytic training at the Inter-Regional Society of Jungian Analysts. Lisa is on the faculty of the Philadelphia Jung Institute. Her writings have appeared in the journal *Psychological Perspectives* and on the blog 4thwavenow. In addition to her analytic practice, Lisa consults with parents whose teens

have self-diagnosed as transgender. She blogs at www.theJungSoul.com
Follow Lisa on Twitter @LisaMarchiano

Susan Matthews
Susan Matthews is an Honorary Senior Research Fellow at the University of Roehampton, UK. She has published widely on histories of gender and sexuality: her 2011 monograph *Blake, Sexuality and Bourgeois Politeness* explores the shifting language of gender and sexuality at the turn of the nineteenth century and shows the ways in which poetic language can challenge gendered concepts. Her current research interests include twentieth century narratives of sex change. Her longer-term project focusses on languages of gender and feeling in an early nineteenth century colonial family. You can follow Susan on Twitter @SusanMatthews

Michele Moore
Michele Moore is a Professor of Inclusive Education and Editor in Chief of the world-leading journal *Disability & Society*. She has worked for more than 30 years in the UK and internationally building research expertise to develop inclusive education and communities. Nowadays her work is focused on consultative participatory human rights and inclusion projects across the world to support children and their families. She has published widely on education, childhood and family life, disability and inclusion. You can follow her on twitter @MicheleMooreEd

Miranda Yardley
Miranda Yardley is a transsexual who has contributed work on freedom of speech and transgender politics to Feminist Current, The New Statesman and The Morning Star, as well as having spoken at many political and feminist events. Miranda's work advocates a materialist, pro-female approach to sex and gender politics that emphasizes compassion, honesty and self-awareness of the consequences of one's own choices and actions. Miranda is by trade an accountant and has published music magazines for the last fifteen years. You can follow Miranda on Twitter @TerrorizerMir

Robert Withers
Robert Withers is a member of the Society of Analytical Psychology, of the BPC and UKCP. He is co-founder of The Rock Clinic in Brighton, UK, where he works as a psychoanalytic psychotherapist and clinical supervisor. He has taught on a number of psychotherapy, counselling and university postgraduate trainings including for the Society of Analytical Psychology and the Inter-university College Graz. His 2015 paper *The*

Seventh Penis, which described some of the difficulties of working psychotherapeutically with people who identify as transgender, recently won the Michael Fordham prize. He also compiled, edited and contributed to the book *Withers*, R. (Ed.) (2003) *Controversies in Analytical Psychology* Routledge Hove and New York. You can follow Bob on Twitter @BobWithers52

CHAPTER ONE

THE FABRICATION
OF 'THE TRANSGENDER CHILD'

HEATHER BRUNSKELL EVANS
AND MICHELE MOORE

People who are broadly liberal and tolerant of gender diversity often fiercely defend adult transgenderism as progressive, even revolutionary. In this view, acceptance of transgenderism means not only support for transgender individuals but for the rights of all gender non-conforming people who belong to the LGBTQI community. Transgender activists who work to normalise transgenderism are admired as bravely working to help steer society away from lingering, old-fashioned bigotry towards the tolerance of 'difference' and acceptance of 'gender fluidity'.

By extension, it is assumed that the practice of transgendering children is equally progressive. It is argued that transgender children are transgender adults in the making whose 'true' 'gender identity' is belied by their external genitalia. For example, a girl can reside in a boy's body, and a boy can be 'trapped' in a girl's body. From this perspective, transgender children have always existed, but have hitherto been denied human rights and social recognition. Nowadays, medicine, social policy, and the law endorse this understanding of 'the transgender child'. Children who do not conform to gender stereo-types and are uncomfortable with their assigned gender are diagnosed as suffering from 'gender dysphoria' – being unhappy in the born body. Gender dysphoria is an alleged medical diagnosis whose treatment includes social gender re-assignment, chemical intervention in puberty if the condition continues, and possibly surgery as a young adult. Support to transition is founded on the belief that children's psychological and physical well-being will be improved, as well as their chances of future happiness and empowerment. Broadcast media have brought transgender children to popular attention, and laud those families who lovingly accept their children's self-defined 'true' gender and support them to transition.

This book is written against the grain of this thinking and practice, and challenges transgender ideology. As Editors, our central contention is that transgender children *don't exist*. Although we argue that 'the transgender child' is a fabrication, we do not disavow that some children and adolescents experience gender dysphoria and that concerned and loving parents will do anything to alleviate their children's distress. It is because of children's bodily discomfort that we argue it is important families and support services are informed by appropriate models for understanding gender. Our analysis of transgenderism demonstrates it is a new phenomenon, since dissatisfaction with assigned gender takes different forms in different historical contexts. The 'transgender child' is a relatively new historical figure, brought into being by a coalition of pressure groups, political activists and knowledge makers. The book examines the theories and politics of transgenderism, and the medical, psychological, legal and educational practices associated with it, for the ways they discursively construct 'the transgender child'.

The book replaces the key concepts of transgender doctrine such as 'non-binary gender' and 'gender as a spectrum'. Bizarrely, in transgender theory, biology is said to be a social construct but gender is regarded as an inherent property located 'somewhere' in the brain or soul or other undefined area of the body. We reverse these propositions with the concept that it is gender, not biology, which is a social construct. From our theoretical perspective, the sexed body is material and biological, and gender is the externally imposed set of norms that prescribe and proscribe desirable behaviours for children. Our objection to transgenderism is that it confines children to traditional views about gender, whereas our vision is that children could be released from binary gender. The norms of gender are not random, but express patriarchal power relations and the pressure to conform to heteronormativity. The sexed body is invested with cultural meaning, so that a girl is induced through social institutions such as the family and school to identify with 'femininity' and a boy is similarly induced to identify with 'masculinity'. If we don't want children and adolescents to be constrained by gender we should be reflexive about embracing it as an inherent, pre-social 'identity' and thus reject the theory of transgenderism.

We are aware that there are different views about transgenderism, some of which are heated, or even publicly disallowed. The purpose of the book is to extend the conversation about transgenderism. Lack of open debate about transgendering children is a casualty of a current culture of offense-taking and identity politics which has had a serious impact on many aspects of free speech. Progressive politics and ethics should surely compel us to reflect upon and discuss theories and practices that may lead to the chemical and surgical transformation of the healthy bodies of children and teenagers. As a society, we are all morally responsible for our young people and, in our view, it is a derogation of our responsibility if, as adults, we did not openly talk about such a serious topic.

In opening up discussion, the contributors to this book have each found that any reflection on transgender doctrine makes us vulnerable to accusations of transphobia, hate speech or of being a Trans-Exclusionary Radical Feminist ('TERF'). We notice that any critique can be inflammatory even to people who are largely disinterested in transgender issues and who are seemingly free from partisan views. We state this reaction at the outset because each of us has been surprised that any reflection on transgenderism, and specifically on 'the transgender child', incurs a unique set of constraints on our voices that we have not experienced in applying a social constructionist methodology to any other area of our academic, clinical or other work to date.

Transgender theory and politics specifically claims transgenderism is a 'gender revolution' which will release children from the oppression of not being allowed to be their 'authentic self'. As Editors, we conclude, that in the guise of offering a new paradigm of thought and a revolution in values, transgendering children is not progressive, but politically reactionary, medically dangerous and abusive of children.

Becoming a community of transcritical thinkers

It seems important at this juncture to describe the process by which concerns about the growing uncritical acceptance of transgender theory and practice of transgendering children evolved. In early 2014, we began researching transgenderism. At this time, we did not know any of the contributors to this book. Our approach to enquiry had led us to begin thinking of ways in which our work on the social construction of gender might critically intervene into emerging knowledges, politics and ethics of transgenderism. To our surprise, our tentative steps towards progressive transcritical thought were responded to as injurious. Heather wrote a post for her University's blog Think Leicester on the social construction of gender and critiquing the celebration by Vanity Fair of the transitioning of Bruce Jenner to Caitlin Jenner as an act of Jenner's bravery in which 'she' had become a 'true' woman (Brunskell-Evans 2015). Formal complaints were made to the University of Leicester including the accusations that

Heather was firstly, being hurtful to possible transgender students and staff and secondly, breaching the 2010 Equality Act. Although these were not upheld we learned a painful lesson that while in most other areas academic research and writing offers a space in which critical thinking can take place, and conflicting theories and opinions can be expressed and debated, on the topic of transgenderism debate is suppressed. We found on this occasion and many since, there is an incredibly high demand for vigilance, policing of speech and a real risk of being silenced. In our experience, transgender activists and their supporters can very quickly falsely accuse transcritical commentators of being oppressive to transgender individuals and of not aspiring to equality.

By the summer of 2015 it was clear that transgender ideology had fired the popular imagination with regards to the rights of transwomen. Submissions were solicited by the Women & Equalities Committee to inform the Transgender Equality Inquiry where written contributions about possible conflict of interests between women and transwomen, were disregarded. At the same time, we became increasingly concerned that unprecedented numbers of children were being identified as transgender and that the practices of transgendering children ran the risk of serious, long-term consequences, medically, psychologically and socially. We realised that public debate was urgently needed where a range of voices could be heard. Questions such as 'Is transgendering children progressive and a sign of a tolerant society?' or 'Is transgendering children potentially harmful and abusive?' were impossible to dialogue in public.

Gradually, through very careful privately conducted conversations often mediated over the internet through false persona, we located allies also struggling to intervene in the trend to diagnose more and more children as transgender. The collection of well-informed careful thinkers we eventually found, working from a range of personal circumstances and experiences, came together in secret in the summer of 2016 from far flung corners of the UK and the USA to discuss transcritical perspectives with the express purpose of protecting children from harm. We came together in fear, making clandestine travel arrangements, each afraid of very real consequences for our families and livelihoods which could arise from our small network of activism. In the safe confines of a sunny board room overlooking a shady metropolitan street we resolved to stand together and reveal our critical concerns through the pages of this book.

And so, in this book the reader will find compelling research-based accounts of central controversies and contentions which underlie the transgendering of children and explain our resistance to identification of children as transgender. Each contributor examines aspects of the personal, political, theoretical, social and cultural impact of transgenderism for children and young people, drawing on their own knowledge and experience. They draw, overtly and implicitly, on a range of personal circumstances to enter the debate from a variety of positions. The contributors bring a wide range of stakeholder perspectives to the debate as academic theorists, practitioners, counsellors, persons living as transgender, persons who have transitioned and regretted it and parents of children and young people identifying as transgender. They analyse transgenderism from their own position of witnessing concern for children and young people to offer a call for critical resistance that contests the current status quo.

The critique of the practice of transgendering children in this book is not aimed personally at any adult who chooses to transition or who has transitioned, at any individual doctor who facilitates the transgendering of children, at any parent who supports their child to transition, and last but not least, at any young person who is thinking about transitioning or is in the process of doing so.

Youth Transcritical Perspectives

In Chapter Two *Stephanie Davies-Arai* Director of Transgender Trend, the leading UK organisation for parents questioning the transgender narrative, outlines the key concepts and questions that have shaped this book. She points to the relationship between growing media coverage of children identified as transgender and the exponential rise in number of children referred to the leading UK Gender Identity Development Service (GIDS). One explanation, she argues, is that the media promulgates the myth that some children are 'born in the wrong body'. This idea is relentlessly promoted by transgender lobbyists within a cultural climate where challenge is silenced. She offers a clue to whose interests the 'transgender child' lobby is really serving by pointing to a change in terminology from 'transsexual' to the euphemism of 'transgender' that obscures the interests of adult lobbyists. She authoritatively dismantles the tyranny of youth transgender suicide statistics, known to be based on falsified data yet routinely used to compel parents to collude in the maintenance of their child's transgender confusion. She exposes the inevitability that falsely exaggerated claims about the incidence of suicide are likely to be driving youth transgender suicide statistics. In contrast to the idea that we are developing increased awareness and sensitivity towards the transgender child, she shows how we are witnessing a new ideology of 'gender identity' which decreases children's freedom as parents and children are induced in clinical and educational settings to believe a single fixed narrative that a child's body can somehow be wrong.

Davies-Arai's analysis makes plain that the increasingly popular trend to transgender children is not benign and easily morphs into homophobic discrimination. She says that "what we have been witnessing is not only a medical experiment on some children's bodies but a psychological experiment on all children's minds". The reader is left questioning whether transgendering children belongs to the world of unreality rather than reality and whether medicine is objective as we might like to believe or is being practiced in Gender Identity Development Services according to a political agenda which has no evidence base that is undermining the health of children and families. There are legitimate common sense questions that must be asked about transgenderism that are crucial to the well-being and safeguarding of children. Davies-Arai makes clear that underpinning the lack of credible reasoning and data to substantiate transgender ideology is deep and purposeful obfuscation of the distinction between sex and gender; this is a theme which contributors to the book make central to analysis of transgender ideology.

In Chapter Three *Heather Brunskell-Evans*, Visiting Research Fellow at Kings' College London, picks up the theme of the social construction of gender and the relationship between medicine and another UK Gender Identity Service, namely Gendered Intelligence which works with children and staff in schools. She explores the power that medicine and Gendered Intelligence have in conveying unproven theories about gender and children to children themselves, to their caretakers and teachers, and to social policy. Firstly, she asks questions of medical knowledge and demonstrates that the medicalized transgendering of children is an individualised response to what is a social issue, namely problems posed by repressive, societal binary gender norms. As such, medicine constructs rather than reveals 'the transgender child'. Secondly, she asks questions of Gendered Intelligence and demonstrates how this organization contributes to the construction of this new, fabricated identity through ideas gleaned from queer theory and an existentialist philosophy of 'choice'. She argues the doctrine of 'non-binary gender' proposed by Gendered Intelligence is intellectually incoherent and confirms rather than subverts gender stereo-types

Brunskell-Evans proposes that when medical practice and organisations such as Gendered Intelligence combine to mobilize children and teenagers to transgender they are not progressive and humane but illiberal and abusive. As such her analysis adds to the conclusion that Davies-Aria draws, namely that transgender theory is mythological and that it is pernicious not only to the individual children who become identified as transgender but to all children in the school communities to which Gendered Intelligence programmes are delivered. In her unequivocal statement that she hopes future generations will look back on the current transgender trend with shame, the reader is charged with the utmost responsibility for making sure they are looking at transgenderism through seeing eyes.

In Chapter Four *GenderCriticalDad* writes as the parent of a trans-identifying teenager. He must remain anonymous to safeguard the confidentiality of his child. His chapter connects the snapshots of the world of transgenderism presented by Davies-Aria and Brunskell-Evans to the actuality of everyday life as the parent of a gender confused teen. He talks about his experience of being on the receiving end of a Gendered Intelligence workshop for teenagers and their parents. He describes his alarm seeing his daughter and other young people in the group exposed to facilitators designated to counsel confused teenagers with no qualifications in education, child development or youth work. The sole determinant of the facilitator's suitability for access to vulnerable young people is that they themselves identify as transgender. In his view, the facilitators showed evident signs of extreme confusions about gender. His disturbing account raises questions about who has influence over our children and young people and who has the power to translate children's expression of gender confusion to transgender ideology.

GenderCriticalDad describes the mundane details of ordinary family life with a teenager, knowing that teenage years can be turbulent, and contrasts this with extra-ordinary narratives provided by transgender doctrine as a means to help them. He talks about his struggle to protect his daughter from untrusted outside influences; he knows his role as a parent is to mitigate and put those influences into a context for his children in order to keep them safe. He illuminates the irony of transgender doctrine which presents parents who question the transgender narrative as the source of unsafe influence on their own children. In desperately wanting to support his daughter and be a good parent he constantly faces the accusation that he is bigoted and transphobic.

GenderCriticalDad finds solace in radical feminist analysis of the distinction made between sex and gender that is completely at odds with transgender theory. A growing number of men understand that radical feminism provides the conceptual tools to interrogate the ideology of transgenderism and to his great surprise GenderCriticalDad is leading the way on this. He is an unlikely candidate for putting his head above the TERF parapet where TERF is the catchall term used to denounce and belittle any radical feminist critique of transgenderism. He explains how parental concern is immediately denounced as being an example of TERF behaviour and oppositional to your own child's best interests. Having read GenderCriticalDad's chapter the reader will be in no doubt about the integrity and reasoning behind his transcritical 'chest full of feelings' that explain the legitimate resistance of any 'parent with a daughter who says she wants to be a man'.

In Chapter Five *Josephine Bartosch*, a feminist activist, explores the coming out stories of women who understood their same sex attraction before transgenderism began to invalidate lesbians. This helps build useful insights into how young people discovering their sexuality can be supported so that their search for a positive sexual identity is not hijacked by discourses of transgenderism. Not surprisingly, all of the women Bartosch talks to remember difficult times during adolescence when their experience of growing up as a female was at odds with stereotypical expectations that govern women's lives, and when they felt under heavy social pressure to modify their feelings, bodies and behaviours to conform to prescribed gender boundaries.

Looking back the women she talked to fear that today's sustained campaign to interpret gender confusion as a sign of being transgender would have put them under considerable pressure at a time when they were self-conscious and already engulfed with confusion. They reflect on the ready deployment of transgender discourses in the lives of young women coming to understand same sex attraction in the current climate as ushering in new forms of oppression, with the prospect of actual bodily harm, and therefore see it as essential to step out of line to challenge the rise of transgender identity politics. Looking back over their shoulders they know their clothes, haircuts, interests and pastimes would have been sufficient to incite and propel definitions of transgender identity – exactly as GenderCriticalDad is witnessing and describes. Bartoch's conversations with the women, and consideration of her own experience, raise serious questions concerning how becoming a lesbian can be powerfully and dangerously disrupted if children and young people fall sufficiently into the gaze of those who are indifferent to the significance of transcritical thinking.

In Chapter Six *Lisa Marciano,* clinical social worker and Jungian analyst, explores the emergence of the fiction of transgender through a Jungian practitioner lens. Her chapter is distinctively different from others in this book because, in contrast to other contributors who focus more directly on political and social factors, she locates transgenderism as an effect of a developmental need of teenagers to discover meaning and to find purpose. In Marciano's view, an eternal adolescent developmental stage is individuation from adult authority by seeking out intense and sometimes dangerous situations. Throughout history young adults have done this by testing themselves whilst belonging to a social group doing the same thing. In the 21st Century she claims this need can be satisfied through the excitement offered by transgender identity as alleged resistance to cultural norms and parental authority. By identifying as transgender teenagers seek to satisfy a universal psychological need for tribal belonging to overthrow parental control. She suggests identifying as transgender is an attempt to "self-initiate, to slip the bounds of banal ordinariness and see meaning and transcendence".

The question may arise of what is wrong with seeking autonomy and independence through transgender doctrine and identification with the transgender community? Marciano argues that irrespective of whatever transgender theory does, or does not contribute to ideas about gender, ultimately its solutions do not reach the roots of what a young person needs. A sensitive appreciation of a young person's need to symbolically transition from teenagehood to adulthood through separation offers a reassuring solution in her chapter that offers connectivity rather than disconnection and difference from others which is integral to transgender explanations of teenagehood. Interventions based on transgender theory may offer, for instance, cosmetic surgery to counteract body dysmorphia but there is evidence that dissatisfaction with the body part altered does not disappear after its physical alteration. In contrast, an appreciation of the symptoms of body dissatisfaction can be resolved through counselling. Taking symptoms of discomfort at the transition from teenage to adulthood at the level of the concrete disclosure by a young person, as transgender theory claims it does, means that we miss the meaning behind the utterances of a young person who is confused about gender. Echoes of arguments presented in all the other chapters of the book can be heard; derogation of responsibility in allowing a developmentally immature person to make decisions that will affect them in their lives in ways which they cannot possibly predict or understand is neither just nor morally comprehensible.

In Chapter Seven *Susan Matthews*, an academic, turns to analysis of the emergence of transgender identity through its construction in literature and storytelling. In contrast to the idea that transgenderism is ahistorical and has been with us forever, she argues that contemporary transgender ideology "is a product of our moment in history, that it invents a new set of beliefs that are without historical precedent". She demonstrates that changes in our understanding of gender can be seen in the "stories produced by novelists, historians, gender theorists, psychiatrists and scientists" taking two sources as the site of her analysis: the 1984 novel The Wasp Factory by Iain Banks which explores genital mutilation in childhood; and the story told by American gender identity specialist John Money in the middle of the 20th century of Bruce Reimer who was accidentally castrated at the age of nine months in a medical accident during circumcision and reassigned as a girl by Money. In this analysis, Matthews argues that 20th century medical technologies have enabled the idea that one can transform the body in to its "real" gender – as if gender was 'real' in contrast to the body which can betray reality.

Matthews further posits that gender has currently taken over from religion as a means of offering escape from distress inherent in the human condition. She shows that in contemporary society all distress is now being referred to the idea of gender disquiet whereas in fact alternatives narratives, seen in the literary examples she explores, suggest alternative routes out of gender distress: we tell ourselves stories to escape unhappiness. Matthews' intent is to decouple the relationship transgender theory makes between unhappiness and gender discontent. What is interesting about The Wasp Factory, Matthews proposes, is that the road to personal and collective freedom will not be built upon gender as key to what is essentially human, but counter-intuitively to a 21st mind, human freedom and happiness can be achieved by recognising the fictional status of gender and thereby releasing us all – adults and children – from gender tyranny.

In Chapter Eight *Carey Callahan* writes as a detransitioned woman interested in alternative treatments for gender dysphoria. Her chapter about her experience detransitioning from a man reads more like poetry than prose. Within the beauty of language and metaphor she conveys the pain and horror of the lies that led her to transition in the first place. She argues that in focusing on her own individual story her chapter does more than illuminate her own life but points also to the "ideological narratives that rule our culture".

In the process of detransitioning Callahan realised that what the transitioning community and modern society spurn is the idea that there is anything about the female body to which one could be loyal. In contrast, loyalty is a performance to the concept of 'femininity' both in the transgender community and in wider society. She longs to abandon the requirement for gender performance and to get back to her own body's experience of the world. The authentic sense of self she longs for is not the one provided for by transgender ideology, namely that she is 'really a man in a woman's body'. It is to return to the authenticity of being a woman in a woman's body and to be allowed to have experiences of that body outside of objectification and the performance of 'femininity'. She wants to have an experience of her body below the level of sexism. In the detransitioning community to which she belonged women were originally on their guard not to bring sexism and objectification of women into their discussion about why women might want to become men for fear that they were letting the trans community down. The transitioning community in fact did reject her and in doing so she felt cast aside like other women throughout the centuries who have been deemed mad, bad or crazy. She notes that discomfort with womanhood takes different forms in different historical contexts: at the time of writing, transitioning to a man is becoming one available way for women to express their discomfort.

Where did the idea of becoming a man to resolve the problems of becoming a woman emerge? Callahan feels feminism let her down in finding alternative ways to be a woman. She turned to Queer feminism which offered liberation from being a 'she'. Queer feminism promised an escape from discomfort with femininity; a promise Callahan learned to her cost could never be realised. It offered her 'gender fluidity' that would let her call herself any pronoun, have sex with every gender in every kind of body. But she discovered the same oppressive feminine roles were just under the surface; what wasn't on offer was any alternative to valuing oneself and one's body on any other basis than the old feminine role of mother or hooker in new disguise. She knows the experience of detransitioners threatens the claims and power of the transitioning community. She refuses to be silenced and will not kowtow to the demands of transgender advocates to render the transregret experience of people like herself invisible. Her radical agenda is for the seldom heard voices of detransitioners to be heard and taken seriously.

Miranda Yardley, a natal man who has chosen to live as a woman, takes Callahan's disappointments with gender ideology further. Yardley now takes an abolitionist stance on gender believing gender damages everyone. He disavows use of the word 'woman' for himself, preferring to use the term 'transsexual'. Yardley describes the rise in children and young people identifying as transgender as a 'modern epidemic' and sets out to answer the question of why we don't respond to this as we would any other new epidemic such as might result from a pathogen, i.e., why don't we attempt to stop the surge of transgenderism rather than support its increase as if it was benign? He reminds us that GIDS openly admits it can find no explanation for the rise in referrals nor can it provide any scientific explanation for gender dysphoria. That gender is a cultural phenomenon is acknowledged by GIDS and the service provides very little understanding of why it is that anyone would be transgender.

In answering the question of why we seem incapable as a society to address this epidemic, Yardley provides two solutions. Firstly, he proposes that pressure not to address the issue comes from transgender lobbyists who are not concerned about children and young people. The concept of 'the transgender child', he reveals, is useful to the transgender lobby and indeed is "central to the campaigning of transgender activism". The transgender activist lobby is aware that to make changes in transgender legislation and gender related language and expression in legislation, transgender identifying youth can be deployed to mobilise support. Using the rights of children and young people to lobby for legislative change is useful because it persuades the movers and shakers of society that transgender is connected to the needs of children and keeping them safe and has nothing to do with the sexual desires of male transvestites.

Secondly, the advancement of scientific knowledge about the aetiology of transgenderism is being obstructed by the same transgender lobbyists "through tactics of threats and intimidation". Scientific enquiry and reporting of it "is tightly politically controlled, in particular, the attacking of any activity seen as being other than affirmative". Research and debate is obstructed through "routine harassment, vilification and intimidation of professionals". Yardley is horrified by this and calls for a change to the cultural climate in which transgenderism can be discussed. He insists there must be scope for rigorous investigation of what it is that makes individuals identify as the opposite sex. Research should be conducted without personal or professional risk and researchers should be free to investigate topics of concern irrespective of political sensitivities, for example, investigating the links between pornography consumption and incitement of sexual pleasure in transgenderism.

Yardley takes up a recurring theme in the book about the role of the media in producing and reproducing affirmative views of transgenderism as a benign, nonthreatening phenomenon. His chapter raises more questions than it answers about the social origins and implications of transgenderism showing there is no room for complacency in relation to the consequences of transgendering children.

In Chapter Ten *Robert Withers*, a psychotherapist whose approach is informed by psychoanalysis, does specifically seek to understand the aetiology of transgenderism. He argues that psychoanalysis can perform that function, and as such, therapy may be able to offer a viable alternative to transgender medical intervention. In his view, it is plausible that "fear of sexuality, dissociation between both mind and body and male and female elements in the personality and issues around identification" may be determinants of gender dysphoria for some of the clients he has worked with. His ideas resonate with those explored by Callahan on possibilities of a relationship between transgender identification and childhood trauma. In contrast to her view that dissociation arises from the cultural constraints of growing up as a girl, Withers describes transgenderism without reference to social context. In his view, transgenderism can be the result of keeping at bay feelings of dissociation arising from childhood trauma and the subsequent fear of being overwhelmed by any resurfacing of them. He suggests it is unsurprising that some people attempt to cope with overwhelming feelings by surgically and hormonally altering their body, but like Callahan, he has been brought directly into contact with people regretting transition.

We saw earlier the scope for transregret experienced by Callahan where transitioning through medical intervention did not alleviate underlying discomfort with living in a female body. However, even finding a clear physical causal explanation for gender dysphoria would not necessarily imply the necessity for medical intervention. The continued failure to provide a biological aetiology for gender dysphoria Withers argues, can only add weight to the importance of psychological or psychotherapeutic rather than medical intervention. He is of course, acutely concerned about accusations of transphobia, finding himself to be operating in a climate where even at professional conferences he attended at the time of writing, transcritical discussion was being decidedly shut down. Not seeking to dodge the difficulty of false accusations of transphobia, Withers ends his chapter by posing the question of whether a therapeutic, psychological approach or a medical approach involving wounding surgery and a lifelong hormone regime best serves people who identify as transgender.

Jen Izaakson is a doctoral candidate with a thought-provoking track record of being asked if she is transgender though she is not. In Chapter Eleven, she proposes the feminism that arises from queer theory, which she calls 'transfeminism', is inadequate for the purposes of challenging an emphatic and self-assured reconceptualization of gender espoused through transgender ideology. A robust engagement with transgender theory is necessary she argues, because academics, psychologists, medical doctors and the public find themselves ill equipped to confront the questions and challenges thrown up by transgender ideology. She seeks to confront the assertiveness of transgender theory and open a space for critical thinking. Theory applied to transgender children she reveals, did not emerge from focus on the physical and well-being of children, but emerged from a focus within the academy on adult sexuality. An interesting aspect of the chapter is Isaacson's views that within the academy the idea of transgenderism has been invented and then researched in ways that seek to demonstrate that it is a naturally occurring phenomenon.

Izaakson says that gender identity theory embedded within transgender doctrine, is a challenge to conventional gender stereotypes. She turns this idea on its head, arguing the converse is true. Both conventional ideas of gender and the key trans concept of 'gender identity' perform a policing of the person. Where conventional gender stereotyping takes the form of objectifying women on the basis that the female body and 'femininity' are the same thing, transgender policing objectifies people by focusing on whether your 'true' gender identity and your body are out of sync. In both cases, whether it is conventional objection or within transfeminism, there is no space for outright refusal of gender and "regulatory gender rules". Once gender identity has become established as something that's 'natural' and 'real' rather than something that is socially constructed then there is a circularity to its logic.

Izaakson argues that clinicians in gender identity clinics do not discuss, and are possibly completely unaware, that they reproduce and act on these confused ideas. Service providers and service users are oblivious to the cycle of transgender construction because firstly it has the appearance of naturalness and secondly, in carrying out their job, they reinforce it. Not only this; clinicians in reproducing transgender in their clinics get caught up in requiring transgenderism as real for their own livelihood. She points to the relationship between transgendering and the financial incentives of the industry (medicine, big pharma etc.) to maintain this illusion.

Finally, *Michele Moore,* Professor of Inclusive Education, argues that transcritical thinking is not oppositional to inclusivity in education and society. She asserts there should be no stigma or discrimination around gender nonconforming children and that responses to a child's gender discomfort must be located in requirement for social change rather than in rejection of a child's body. She sees gender discomfort as located in social injustice which has to be tackled through social change – not through intervention that compromises children's the integrity of bodies. She points out that entitlements of children and young people to self-determination are being drowned out by dominant voices of transgender activists, especially in schools. Far from promoting well-being and social justice, powerful institutions upholding transgender ideology are taking away freedoms, eroding respect for individuality that is the foundation stone for inclusion and acceptance in all spheres of life and, at the same time, annihilating the physical and mental health of unprecedented numbers of children and young people. Her analysis exposes transgender activism as having hugely restrictive implications for children's rights to self-expression. She draws parallels between the current fashion for intervention on children's healthy bodies and treatment systems for disabled children that have come and gone in different historical contexts to show that critical voices must be sustained in the face of movements that seem to promise liberation but neglect to adequately face up to possible harms. She concludes that a sign of a truly progressive society is one where serious critical debate can take place and that the contributors of this book work toward such a society.

And so, at the end of this book the reader will have engaged with many arguments about the importance of critical intervention in the seemingly unstoppable celebration of transgender ideology in the lives of children and young people. We advocate adherence to the principle of First, Do No Harm. There is constant abreaction to the analyses of all contributors to this book which has not deterred us but, in contrast, has strengthened our resolve to address the phenomenon of transgendering children. The authors call for an open debate about the divide between gender confusion and intervention. We argue that if discussion of any topic is silenced or shut down through personal slurs or name-calling this is probably the very moment at which we should open it to further critical scrutiny. This book is the result of our collective persistent questioning.

CHAPTER TWO

THE TRANSGENDER EXPERIMENT ON CHILDREN

STEPHANIE DAVIES-ARAI

In April 2015 an episode of the popular Louis Theroux series, entitled 'Transgender Kids' was broadcast on BBC2 (Theroux, 2015). Although media coverage of the subject had already been steadily growing in the UK, this was probably the moment when the issue of 'transgender kids' was brought into full mainstream awareness. The number of children referred to the Tavistock gender clinic in London over that year doubled. Concurrent with increasing media coverage, the Tavistock clinic has seen an increase in referrals of nearly 1000% over the past six years (BBC News, 2016). Each year has seen a 50% increase in referrals and during that time the number of children less than ten years of age has increased four-fold. The reversal in the sex ratio since 2009/10, when figures were first recorded, has been expanding year on year and the number of girls is now nearly double that of boys: 913 out of the 1,398 children and adolescents referred in 205/16. The average age of referral was fourteen.

One simple story has been popularised to explain this unprecedented increase in numbers: that some children are 'born in the wrong body' and that it is the increased public awareness and acceptance of transgender people which has inevitably led to a greater number of children and adolescents who feel able to 'come out' as transgender. What this explanation fails to acknowledge is that a single fixed narrative, that of 'courageous children daring to be their authentic selves and the brave parents who support them' has been relentlessly promoted to the public within a climate where any challenge has been silenced by accusations of hatred and bigotry (Banned by Trans, undated) and all debate shut down (Transgender Trend, 2016).

It is not only 'increased awareness' we have been witnessing but a sustained campaign to promote a new ideology of 'gender identity' which persuades parents that their child's body is 'wrong' and teaches children that 'sex is between your ears and not between your legs'. Quietly, the idea that sterilising children by blocking their natural sexual development (Mirror.co.uk, 2011) and then medically altering their healthy bodies with synthetic cross-sex hormones, followed by possible surgery and lifelong risky medication, has been accepted as the new orthodoxy (Taylor, 2015).

Girls will be boys and boys will be girls

Through exploiting confusion in the public mind between 'sex' (the biological reality of being male or female) and 'gender' (the social idea of masculine and feminine), transgender organisations have managed to mask the inherent contradictions of a reactionary ideology. The fact that changing your sex to match your 'gender identity' reinforces the very stereotypes which these organisations claim to be challenging is effectively hidden in plain sight as, in increasing numbers, boys who love princess culture become 'girls' and short-haired football-loving girls become 'boys'.

Promoted as a 'progressive' social justice movement based on 'accepting difference', transgender ideology in fact takes that difference and stamps it out. It says that the sexist stereotypes of 'gender' are the true distinction between boys and girls and biological sex is an illusion. In this ideology, 'being feminine' has replaced being female as the very definition of 'girl'.

The sympathetic story of helping children to become 'who they really are', together with the change in terminology from 'transsexual' to 'transgender', has worked to sanitise the story and obscure the reality. A diagnosis previously reserved for adults may now be applied to children with little resistance from parents, not many of whom would be comfortable with the label 'transsexual' for their child. It is hard to imagine a parent at the school gate saying of their six year-old 'this is my daughter Chloe, she's transsexual'.

Transition or die

An integral part of the celebratory media story has been the darker supporting narrative of the inevitable suicide outcome if children are not supported in their transition. If parents need one more push to believe the new ideology, this is the one that does it. With no evidence that treatment cures suicidal ideation (nor recognition that hormonal drugs, as a side-effect, may exacerbate it), transgender youth support organisations such as

Mermaids regularly broadcast the threat to worried parents and a gullible media (Kleeman, 2015).

From parents in media interviews we typically hear 'I want a happy daughter, not a dead son'. Children get taught the script and the media has eagerly given them a platform to spread the message: a 16-year-old talking on the BBC Radio 4 programme Beyond Binary (BBC Analysis, 2016) says that if she couldn't transition "I would probably kill myself." The Guardian, in an article about sex-reassignment surgery describes it as "life-saving work" (Lyons, 2016).

We have never before taught children they can decide their sex; this is an experiment. Let's see how it's going.

The creation of the transgender child

The medical term for the condition in which someone feels discomfort or distress in their sexed body is 'gender dysphoria'. However, Louis Theroux's programme was not entitled 'Gender Dysphoric Kids' and nowhere across the media do we hear any word other than 'transgender' used to describe these children. The actual definition of the term (National Centre for Transgender Terminology, 2014) is "a person whose gender identity is different from the sex they were assigned at birth" as though your sex is something randomly decided by strangers. Calling a child 'transgender' in fact signifies nothing other than allegiance to the belief that a child's gender identity *is* their true sex.

In using the term 'transgender kids' it is not the kids we are protecting and advocating for, but the ideology itself. More sinisterly, the word is used by transgender organisations as an umbrella term for all so-called 'gender questioning', 'gender non-conforming' and 'gender variant' children, thus sweeping up all children who don't conform 100% to stereotype. The 'transgender' label treats all 'gender dysphoric' children as a homogenous group; the reason an infant boy who loves playing with dolls believes he is really a girl becomes exactly the same reason a troubled autism spectrum teenage girl thinks she is really a boy: 'because they are transgender'. An adult identity politics has been applied to children and young people whose identities are not fixed but are in a process of being built through experience and interaction with the environment; identities which are highly vulnerable to influence from adults.

A new way to be homophobic

The overwhelming majority of children who experience gender dysphoria will not carry those feelings into adulthood (around 80% desist) (Cantor, 2016) and most of those children, if left alone, will turn out to be gay, lesbian or bi-sexual as adults (Bailey and Zucker, 1995). There is no reliable method of discerning which children will persist and which won't: to apply any rigid essentialist theory to highly suggestible young children can only create a self-fulfilling prophecy and effectively operates as a new form of gay conversion therapy.

Neither parents nor children live in a cultural bubble, immune to any influence from society. The fact that at a very young age boys outnumber girls, but teenage girls vastly outnumber teenage boys at the Tavistock clinic, in itself demonstrates the existing social influence behind those referrals. Societal acceptance of 'tomboys' versus relative hostility towards young boys who express 'girly' interests must play some part in parents' readiness to believe their little boys are transgender but not so much their girls. Parents who in the past may have forced a 'macho' role onto sons they feared were homosexual, now have a socially-sanctioned way to 'stamp out the gay'.

For girls, adolescence is the time when they are suddenly expected to live up to impossible ideals of femininity, a time when approval is withdrawn for any 'boyish' behaviour or appearance they managed to get away with when young. It is not surprising that this is a time of 'sudden onset gender dysphoria' for girls. Defining themselves as 'straight guys' becomes an attractive option for teenage lesbians within a society which views lesbians as either failed women or a male pornographic fantasy. While a 'trans' identity is accepted and cool, 'lezza' is still the worst insult thrown at a girl in school. We need to tackle lesbophobia as a distinct category based on both homophobia and misogyny if we want to support these girls; transgender orthodoxy just enables us to look the other way.

For a new idea to take root and grow, the existing culture must provide a fertile soil. Transgender orthodoxy has landed in a society already primed to accept the idea that girls can be boys, and boys girls, and that it's time we let children choose.

Sexist stereotypes

We have never trained children into such extreme stereotyped sex-roles from birth as we have done over the last decade (Sweet, 2014). Through industry marketing designed to maximise profits, the toys, books and clothes produced for children today, as never before, shoehorn boys into the blue box and girls into the pink box, with no room for overlap.

A belief in sexist stereotypes has been fostered for decades, particularly through media sexual objectification of women (Hatton and Trautner, 2011) as well as books like *Men Are from Mars, Women Are from Venus* (at the time of writing still the biggest-selling self-help book of all time). The message reinforced through both print and broadcast media is that men and women are different species, women valued primarily for how they look and men for what they do. These are the messages that influence us all and which children imbibe every day through our image-saturated public culture.

No matter that brain research shows us that male and female brains are far more alike than they are different and that many of the stereotypes we cherish are simply not true (Fine, 2013), the cultural messages all around us say the opposite. When a little boy who prefers playing with Barbie dolls looks around him today, the message he gets everywhere, in toy shops, toy packaging, advertising (Peck, 2015) and perhaps from his parents, is that only girls play with Barbie, so it is easy to see how childish logic could tell him "I must be a girl." If we define the gender boxes for children so rigidly, it is not surprising that a child who does not fit into the one designated for their sex might see no alternative but to join the other one; we give children no space to exist comfortably between the two extremes. How much is a child's 'gender identity' formed by internalisation of these cultural messages that children are bombarded with every day?

The self-knowing child

The 'innate gender identity' theory also feeds into an idea already established in the parenting advice industry. A 'child-led' parenting model based on the tenets of 1950s attachment theory has gained traction over the last few decades, reflecting the wider societal shift to a politics of personal identity rights. The sub-text of child-centred parenting suggests that children know who they are, they know themselves best and they are born with a fully-developed self, the expression of which it is the parent's job to enable. One of the central skills of child-centred parenting is that of listening to the child and centring their feelings. Listening is very easily conflated with 'agreeing' in this 'child-knows-best' model. It is easy to see how a child's feelings can quickly become consolidated as the strongest reality in a child's mind when they are afforded such central importance by a parent. Comments of parents of 'transgender kids' in media reports invariably reflect this tenet of modern parenting; 'I just listened to him, he knows who he is, he knows himself best'. These parents are not unusual in their belief in their child's level of self-knowledge. But a four year-old can only know themselves as a four year-old, just as a 15 year-old can only know who they are as a teenager: children, by definition, are unable to countenance themselves ever changing. Nowhere do we see society's concordance with this view of children more clearly than in the new responsibility we are giving them to decide their sex, handing over authority to children on a matter they cannot possibly fully understand until their psychosexual development is complete.

For parents, the two beliefs - a child is a gender stereotype, born with a fully developed self-identity - remain unshaken as long as a child chooses toys from the right box. If they choose from the 'wrong' box, however, these two ideas are in conflict. A 'girl in a boy's body' is a neat theory which allows parents to reconcile two beliefs they may hold dear. There exists no media story of 'trans kids' in which a parent does *not* cite toy or clothes preferences as evidence that their child is really the opposite sex. The idea of 'transgender kids' is just an extension of pre-existing ideas; a logical conclusion in a world where children are seen as fully autonomous mini-adults with identities impervious to influence, and who come ready-made in two varieties, pink or blue.

Nevertheless, for a new belief to achieve mass acceptance it takes serious work. What we have been witnessing is a concerted campaign to enforce this ideology throughout the media, schools, public organisations and government. To explain the phenomenal rise in referrals to gender clinics, we need to know exactly what the message is that is being sent to children and young people and how they are likely to understand it.

Children's teatime TV

As children typically outgrow gender dysphoria, the Endocrine Society advises against full social transition of pre-pubertal children (Hembree et al, 2009). Nevertheless, the BBC has promoted social transition as both positive and normal directly to young children themselves (Transgender Trend, 2016a). 'I Am Leo' was a documentary first shown in 2014 on CBBC, a channel aimed at an audience of six to twelve year-olds. Through the programme primary school age children are informed "Leo was born as Lily but has lived as a boy since the age of five". Leo, the audience of children are told, now loves "beat-boxing and doing all the things a 13-year-old boy would normally do. What makes Leo different is that he was born with a girl's body. He has become one of the first children in Britain to be prescribed hormone blockers to prevent him growing into a young woman".

The message is hammered home through an animation which shows a row of figures being sprayed pink and another row sprayed blue on a kind of conveyor belt of production of girls and boys. The pink girls then have pink brains added and the blue boys get blue ones. Those pink girls who don't feel very 'girly' then have blue brains added and the blue boys who don't feel very 'macho' get pink brains. These children are not ordinary children with a normal range of interests, but 'transgender'.

Visually, what better way to teach children that gender stereotypes are the immutable reality: a girl here is redefined as 'a person who is 100% feminine' and a boy becomes 'someone who is 100% masculine'. The animation both pathologises the child who defies stereotype and normalises the 'transgender' child. Leo personalises and embodies this new truth in a way that children can relate to and the documentary presents a simple medical solution.

The CBBC reinforced the message further with a fictional account of a boy becoming a 'girl' in their 2016 web drama Just A Girl which "follows a young girl telling the story of her transition". The character of 11 year-old 'Amy' is played by an actress, a double deception suggesting that the BBC know that the reality of an actual boy playing the part of a girl would provoke some unease in children at the age of puberty, not to mention their parents. A BBC spokesman defended the drama (Gill, 2016) by stating that the fictional transgender character was "trying to make sense of the world, deal with bullying and work out how to keep her friends, which are universal themes that many children relate to" – a defence which offers nothing but the perfect template to manipulate children into accepting a message.

The story of the misfit is a universal one: what child who is bullied or isolated for being 'different' would not recognise themselves in these stories of kids who struggle to fit in with their peer group? CBBC could have made a programme about how societal gender stereotypes hold us back from being the boy or girl we really want to be. But with no other explanation offered, and having never commissioned a documentary about gay, lesbian or bi-sexual young people, the message CBBC sends to children is that if you don't fit in with your same-sex peers you are 'transgender'.

Re-education in Primary schools

Taking 'sex' out of the equation through use of the term 'transgender' has allowed transgender organisations to get the idea into primary schools before the age at which we start talking to children about homosexuality. It gives transgender ideology a head start in influencing children before they have had a chance to grow up, mature sexually, and come to the realisation that they are actually gay or lesbian. Gendered Intelligence is one such activist organisation which visits UK primary schools (Sanchez Manning, 2015) delivering assemblies and workshops to children as young as four.

The Gender Identity Research and Education Society (GIRES) has called for children to be taught about 'atypical gender identity development' in the curriculum from the age of three (Spillet, 2015). Teaching children that it is fine to be 'atypical' simply involves allowing children to play with whatever they want, encouraging all children in an expansive definition of who they can be, and having no tolerance for any teasing or bullying of those children whose behaviour does not fit the stereotype for their sex. What GIRES and other transgender organisations are advocating however, is giving children the opposite message: if you are a boy who likes what society deems to be 'girl' interests the only explanation is that you are really a girl.

At three to five years of age children are at the stage of development when their understanding of the sexes is based on stereotypes of superficial appearance and interests. This is the age of magical thinking; the belief that you can make life anything you want it to be (Miller, et al, 2017). Transgender ideology makes absolute sense to children at this immature developmental stage of understanding. It is between the ages of five and six that children begin the important developmental step of learning to distinguish between fantasy and reality. From this age children are also starting on a path of maturation out of their stereotyped beliefs about the sexes; they are learning that 'boy' and 'girl' are categories with stable properties which do not change according to how you behave or what you wish for.

If we pull the rug of reality out from under little children by teaching them that boys and girls are not in fact stable categories but abstract ideas, we strike at the heart of all children's security in an area fundamental to how they understand themselves. We have no idea of the developmental impact on children who are taught that a boy or a girl has fewer recognised characteristics than a table - in fact none at all, it is just about personal feelings.

Children believe adults. The parents who followed the suggestion in Brighton & Hove City Council's schools' admission form (Wadsworth, 2016) to "support your child to choose the gender they most identify with" would be giving their children a very strong message: you can choose if you're a boy or a girl, it depends on how you feel. Any girl who rejects dolls in favour of rough and tumble play may identify *with* the boys she plays with; it takes one more push for her to identify *as* one of those boys and this push is coming from adults. Teaching young children that their 'authentic self' is disassociated from the body actively trains children into a mind-body split, recognised as a state of dis-ease within health practice, but in this case, uniquely, recast as a psychologically healthy state.

'Prevention of bullying'

In 2016 the Department for Education launched a £2 million grant programme to prevent 'homophobic, bi-phobic and transphobic bullying' in schools, an increasingly common way of teaching transgender ideology to schoolchildren through LGBT support initiatives. Of course, children were not bullied at school for being 'transgender' until we started calling them that. The fact that the routine bullying of children who defy gender and sex-role stereotypes is rooted in homophobia and sexism is effectively disguised by calling it 'transphobia'. Calling non-conforming children 'transgender' not only covers up the real issues of homophobia and sexism which are still rife in schools, but serves to validate those underlying attitudes. A little boy is mocked by being called a 'girl' and transgender ideology supports the bullies: he is a girl. Once he 'becomes' a girl there is no longer anything to mock and the bullies have won. Nine year old Poppy, commenting on BBC Radio 4's Today programme sums up the inherent reinforcement of the bullies' message:

> "Something felt wrong inside. I didn't feel like myself. I didn't feel right. They made fun of me so I changed to a girl and they like me more now, they like me as I am."
> (BBC Today, 2016)

Is this seriously what we are advocating as part of bullying prevention in schools?

For secondary school pupils, the Crown Prosecution Service provides a comprehensive teaching resource on 'LGBT bullying prevention' (Crown Prosecution Service, undated) which explicitly threatens adolescents with hate crime charges if they do not comply in obeying the new doctrine of gender identity. Using activist materials, this resource frames any valid discomfort girls may feel about males in their toilets and changing-rooms as 'prejudice, discrimination and hate'. It omits information about current sex-based rights and protections for girls, the very group who are facing unprecedented levels of sexual harassment and abuse across UK schools (Commons Select Committee, 2016). At the age of sexual development when girls are at their most vulnerable, they are told they have no right to their own boundaries as a sex; that they must protect the feelings of a male classmate above their own need for privacy, comfort and psychological safety. Teaching 'consent' in schools is meaningless if girls are given no right to *not* consent to males in their private spaces if those males 'identify' as female. By aligning the 'T' with 'LGB', girls who complain are painted not only as 'transphobic' but 'anti-LGBT rights'. It is not just the threat of punishment by law which will frighten and shame girls into submission, but the fear of being ostracised from their peer group at the age when belief in social justice causes is at its most passionate.

The schools toolkit

The Transgender Schools Toolkit (Allsortsyouth, 2014) has become a staple of transgender organisations, LGBT groups and local councils across the UK. The GIRES lesson plan (Gires, 2017) echoes CBBC's animation in its portrayal of pink-brained girls and blue-brained boys, in contravention of all NUT guidelines designed to tackle those very stereotypes. Transgender school resources typically begin with a disingenuous claim of 'supporting gender diversity' followed seamlessly by information about 'being transgender'. The obfuscating language typical of these teaching resources effectively covers up the real message sent to children: that if you are in any way 'diverse' you are 'trans'. This is not just misinformation but dangerously misleading for children who, once taught to define themselves as 'trans', are then encouraged along the now established path of invasive and irreversible medical treatment.

A guidebook called *Can I Tell You about Gender Diversity* (Transgender Trend, 2016b) distributed by the government-funded organisation Educate and Celebrate, endorsed by Ofsted, is described by the publishers as "the first book to explain medical transitioning for children aged seven and above". What is the message of this publication? Being 'diverse' requires medical intervention; effectively for example, if you are a gender non-conforming boy you must be made into a girl. The guidebook in reality teaches the opposite of what it pretends: gender diversity will not be tolerated; everyone will be made to conform.

The conflation of 'sex' and 'gender' welds 'female' to 'feminine' and 'male' to 'masculine' so that 'smashing the gender binary' means not that males can be feminine, but that males must literally change to females and vice versa, creating an association between the physical sexed body and the concept of non-conformity in children's minds. Thus children are deliberately misled into recasting 'feminine personality traits' as 'female gender identity'. Children who don't feel themselves to be 100% masculine or feminine are placed literally somewhere between biologically male and female, accounting for a growing number of young people who previously would not have thought to label themselves at all. The result of this belief was demonstrated on the BBC Radio 4 programme 'I'm a Non-Binary 10-Year-Old' (BBC iPM, 2016) by Leo who stated:

> "No, I'm not a boy or a girl. I'm non-binary, so I'm in the middle. There isn't a body of the two genders. I just wish there was some way in the middle. But I don't think there is."

It is only transgender doctrine which misleads young people into thinking that some personality traits are literally 'male' or 'female' and that your body must match your personality. Non-binary is a growing category and double mastectomy increasingly the surgery of necessity for 'enbies' who are girls. Leo is astute in her observation that it is her breasts which will cause the biggest problem later, as they are the most visible indication that she is female.

A new way for girls to self-harm

Collusion in reproducing the harmful ideas outlined above was illustrated in guidelines issued by Local Authorities in Cornwall, Lancashire and Scotland to allow 'transgender pupils' extra breaks during physical education lessons because "some youngsters who choose to bind their chests may suffer from breathing difficulties and fainting" (Sandman, 2016). The sex-neutral 'transgender' category hides the fact that it is only girls who are binding their breasts, denying adolescent girls the support which recognises their unique problems and needs.

The harms of binders are documented in a 2015 study (Peitzmeier et al, 2017) which indicates 28 potential negative outcomes, including compressed or broken ribs, punctured or collapsed lungs, back pain, compression of the spine, damaged breast tissue, damaged blood vessels, blood clots, inflamed ribs and even heart attacks. The necessity for shallow breathing in itself restricts the flow of oxygen to vital organs resulting in a restriction in physical activity harmful to overall health. A mother speaking on Radio 4's Bringing Up Britain programme explained her response to her daughter's double mastectomy as "relief" that she had "got her lungs back" after a year wearing a binder.

Any other practice of self-harm is recognised as such but these Local Authority guidelines declare binders as very important for girls' 'psychological well-being'. Refusal to recognise binders as damaging contrasts with condemnation of similarly harmful practices of other cultures such as breast ironing (Dearden, 2015). To say that girls 'choose' binders absolves us of the responsibility to question the ideology which has created that 'choice' and to question whether we should be teaching and encouraging it in schools.

The erasure of girls

Girls are further made invisible by the increasing adoption of so-called 'gender neutral' language in schools as urged by transgender organisations. Gendered Intelligence, for example, advised the Girls' Schools Association to stop calling girls 'girls' in assemblies in case any girls 'identify' as boys. This is not 'gender neutral' but a de-sexing of language which, as we see in the wider culture, works only to erase the word 'woman' (Donnolly, 2017). Effectively we are educating girls into the class that dare not speak its name.

In adopting a policy which recognises that "your gender is a choice" St. Paul's Girls' School in west London reinforces to girls that being a certain way (having short hair? having an interest in gaming but no interest in fashion?) makes you a boy (Topping, 2017). The policy tells girls that being a 'girl' is an option, not a fact of biology, thus indoctrinating girls into the idea that boys can also be girls if they feel like it and girls must accept them as such. Yet 'girl' is not a subjective idea, it is a fact and it means 'young female'. There are infinite ways of being a girl, none of which tip you over into being a boy. Girls' schools fail in their duty to girls by buying into this new pressure on those who don't conform to stereotype to redefine themselves as boys, and the teachers at girls' schools, of all people, should be resisting the sexist assumptions behind it.

Adolescent identities

Adolescence is a crucial period of identity development as teenagers do the important job of figuring themselves out as they move from childhood to adulthood. This is a long process of exploration; the adolescent brain does not reach full maturity until around age 25 and even as adults our self-identities develop and change. Teenagers have never before been taught that it is normal and necessary to define their personalities in terms of 'gender' when building their self-identities.

The confusion we are creating for adolescents was illustrated by a Gender Survey for 13-15-year-olds, commissioned by the Children's Commissioner and sponsored by the Department for Education, sent out to schools in 2016 (Doughty, 2016). It included a question encouraging teenagers to pick their 'genders' from a list which included 'boy' and 'girl' as 'identity' choices in amongst a whole raft of more interesting alternatives. The message to teenagers is clearly that ticking the 'girl' option is an admission that you conform to stereotypical femininity unless you also tick one of the other options such as 'non-binary' to show that you don't. Getting girls who are uncomfortable with femininity to define themselves as one of the other categories is the first step on the road to questioning whether they are really girls at all. If girl now means 'stereotypical girl' then they are clearly not.

Porn culture and the girls who don't want to be women

In teaching children and adolescents that your sex is a personal choice, we find that it is overwhelmingly teenage girls who have caught the ball and are running with it (Transgender Trend, 2016c). There is now a pattern emerging in secondary schools where girls are 'transitioning' in clusters. The proportion of girls who are suffering co-existing mental health disorders is noted to be significantly increasing at the Tavistock gender clinic (Transgender Trend, op cit).

There is a mental health crisis amongst young people generally, but the group suffering most is adolescent girls and young women (Campbell, 2016). In 2007 the American Psychological Association published its report on the sexualisation of girls (APA, 2007) which was followed by a government-commissioned study entitled Sexualisation of Young People (Papadopoulis, 2010). This latter study foresaw the spread of mainstream pornography through the rise in new technologies and its damaging effects on the health of young girls, as well as the rise in assaults against them. The symptoms in adolescent girls noted in both studies are not dissimilar to the co-existing disorders observed in teenage girls with 'sudden onset gender dysphoria' at the time of writing: lack of confidence in, and comfort with, own body, disassociation, shame, anxiety, self-disgust, low self-esteem, depression, negative mood, eating disorders, negative body image and sense of self, self-objectification and self-harming behaviours.

In her oral evidence to the UK government Transgender Equality Inquiry in September 2015 Dr Bernadette Wren, Associate Director of the Tavistock clinic, observed that "a much higher proportion of natal females is coming forward who have got through to puberty but who now really dislike their female body". Wren continued: "I have to see that in the context of the attack on female bodies and the general sense that feminism has not delivered" but this point was not explored further, nor was it referenced in the Women and Equalities Committee's subsequent report in December 2015.

The difference between the time of writing, and the period 2007-10 when the two previously mentioned reports were published, is that violent porn culture has expanded even further into the lives of young people. Sexual harassment and assault of girls in schools has reached epidemic proportions, and girls have been presented with a brand-new model of interpretation of their feelings, together with an instant solution and route of escape. Society has primed girls to see their own bodies as 'wrong', to view them as objects in need of changing: disassociation from the physical body has already been created, along with girls' sense of failure and self-blame. It's not a huge jump from the body-modification attempts girls already make to the idea of synthetic hormones, breast-binding and mastectomy (Davey, 2016). As long as society continues to objectify and dehumanise women, we must expect to see more vulnerable girls wanting to opt out of womanhood altogether: this group represents a market in waiting for transgender activists.

Social contagion

In our refusal to look at the culture in which our girls are growing up, we can assume that girls are happily immune to any harmful cultural messages and experiences. We can also remain blind to the direct influences on teenage girls through social media platforms such as Tumblr and Reddit, and we fail to see the typical pattern for adolescent girls to 'come out' as transgender after bingeing on these sites (4thWaveNow, 2016).

The BBC Radio 4 programme Beyond Binary casually referenced the role of the internet as 'crucial' in influencing young people to adopt a transgender identity. Jen Jack Giesking, a New York based academic, stated: "there really isn't a trans person I've met under the age of 30 who hasn't been significantly affected by the kind of images they've seen there" (BBC, 2016 op cit). We recognise the phenomenon of social contagion through online sites which glorify harmful behaviours such as cutting, eating disorders and suicide, and we know that teenage girls are the group most active in the world of social media and particularly susceptible to the influence of these sites. Yet online transgender forums and YouTube videos (Transgender Reality, 2016) which encourage young people onto a medicalised 'trans' path are not considered harmful and 'social contagion' cannot even be recognised within an ideology of hard-wired identity which is, by definition, immune to societal influence.

The betrayal of autism spectrum children

One of the most shocking aspects of the exponential rise in referrals to the Tavistock gender clinic is that 50% of the children sent there exhibit autism spectrum traits (Transgender Trend, 2016d). No adolescent is mature enough to understand that they are being indoctrinated into identity and 'queer' politics, nor able to predict the reality of a lifetime on this medical path, which even the 'gender specialists' don't know. Autism spectrum adolescents, who struggle to understand social rules, are particularly vulnerable to the literal thinking behind the idea that if you have feminine personality traits you are a girl, and especially susceptible to the rigid thinking which will keep them stuck in a 'trans' identity once they have been taught to define themselves as such. In a case illustrated on the Channel 4 documentary Kids on The Edge: The Gender Clinic (Channel 4, 2016) the key factor in the development of a 'trans' identity for autistic adolescent Matt, was the bullying from classmates because of Matt's inability to correctly perform a 'feminine' gender role. Matt is forced to make a choice between two gender stereotypes and chooses the one that best fits: a boy. Thus, bullied for not conforming morphs into bullied for being 'trans'.

Teachers are now disabled in their ability to protect children diagnosed as on the autism spectrum and all other special needs children, along with those who are troubled or have experienced previous trauma or sexual abuse, because transgender orthodoxy demands that they immediately accept a child's new identity at face value. Even the most vulnerable groups of children are not exempt from the rule. Transgender orthodoxy itself prevents us from asking any questions.

Recruitment into a cult?

The effect of indoctrinating children into this new gender orthodoxy is becoming apparent. During 2015-16, the number of children seeking counselling about gender identity from the NSPCC's helpline Childline more than doubled (Kirby, 2016) with 2,796 calls made compared with 1,299 calls the previous year: an average of eight calls a day. If these children were looking for adults to help them with gender confusion, all they will get from Childline counsellors is yet more indoctrination because a child's questions about being transgender must be routinely accepted as evidence of being transgender (Childline, undated). There is in fact no escape: child protection agencies, therapists and counsellors, teachers, all are being told that anything less than 'affirmation of preferred gender' is 'conversion therapy'. As a society we are systematically dismantling any means of support or access to any model of understanding for children who are struggling with gender issues other than transgenderism.

While parents are directed towards support groups such as Mermaids, children may be directed towards one of over 250 youth transgender support groups across the UK. All these organisations will do is validate and reinforce a transgender identity and provide vulnerable adolescents with the 'tribe' they were looking for. Any teenager who previously struggled to fit in will find, perhaps for the first time, approval and belonging in these groups, as long as they identify as transgender. Some organisations will even provide camping trips where teenagers can really bond over a shared 'trans' identity (Gendered Intelligence, 2017). There are no other support groups for children and young people who feel they don't 'fit in' because of gender confusion; transgender organisations have the monopoly on these vulnerable teens. The period of adolescence is characterised by risky behaviour, poor decision-making and inability to weigh up long-term consequences or make accurate benefit and risk calculations. The most vulnerable and troubled teenagers are especially ill-equipped to protect themselves from the influence of organisations whose modus operandi looks more like the recruitment tactics of a cult than genuine support for confused young people.

The true agenda of transgender support organisations was hinted at during an interview conducted with Susie Green, CEO of Mermaids on BBC2's Newsnight programme in 2016. The evidence across all published studies is that the percentage of children who outgrow gender dysphoria is around 80%. According to Green however, the desistance rate for children with gender dysphoria amongst over 800 families who sought support from Mermaids is inexplicably much lower "I've probably seen about six" she claimed.

The end of safe-guarding and duty of care

At the time of going to print 'gender identity' is not yet enshrined in law as the definitive distinction between men and women as the Women and Equalities Committee has proposed, but schools, child protection agencies, public organisations and social services are already acting as if it is an established truth.

Girl Guiding UK continues to promote itself as an organisation for girls only, their stated mission: "We give girls a space just for them. We're girls only. That means girls feel free to be themselves" (Girl Guiding, undated). Only on the Diversity and Equality page of their website is their deception of girls revealed, in the declaration of "support for all children and young people who self-identify as a girl or young woman and for adults who self-identify as a woman".

Redefining 'girl' and 'woman' as self-identities takes away any distinction between males and females and erases all safe-guarding policies for girls. Adolescent and adult males are not only granted a new socially-sanctioned means to access girls' private spaces, including on camping and overnight trips, but girls are denied the right to recognise or name them as males. The grooming of young girls to allow the violation of their boundaries puts them at further risk throughout their lives, as they are systematically coached into ignoring their own intuition and warning signals, through fear of hurting the feelings of males.

Transgender ideology demands policies which allow for no recognition of biological sex. The most vulnerable girls in our society, such as those in institutional care homes, are especially at risk of exploitation by any predatory male who now has a fail-safe way to gain access to their private spaces, unfettered by local authorities who would not dare challenge his 'gender identity'. Just as the 'affirmation only' rule substitutes obedience to an orthodoxy for normal duty of care principles in the treatment of 'trans'-identified children, so the 'gender identity' rule substitutes a 'trust all men' approach in place of secure safe-guarding protocols for all girls and young women.

A medical experiment

The most glaring contradiction of an incoherent transgender ideology can be seen in its claims that although sex is irrelevant to whether you are a boy or a girl, it is your biological sex characteristics which must be prevented from developing and then cosmetically altered. The stakes are high: if children take blockers in early puberty and progress to cross-sex hormones at the age of sixteen they will be sterilised as gametes have not had a chance to mature (Boghani, 2015). It is the flood of sex hormones at puberty which triggers the enormous changes in the adolescent brain and it is not known whether interrupting this process prevents full maturation of the frontal lobe functions which develop from puberty until the mid-twenties (Blakemore et al, 2010).

We are already hearing of the devastating effects on the long-term health of women who were prescribed these blockers for precocious puberty (Scutti, 2013) and yet the Tavistock has been prescribing their off-label use for 'transgender kids' since 2011. The use of synthetic cross-sex hormones - testosterone for girls, estrogen for boys - has only recently been tried on children so young. We don't know the effects of synthetic cross-sex hormones on young developing bodies or of the cumulative effects over a lifetime's use: children prescribed these treatments are guinea-pigs (Jewett, 2017). The documented adverse outcomes for men using synthetic versions of testosterone include heart attack, heart failure, stroke, depression, hostility, aggression, liver toxicity, personality changes and infertility (Fox, 2016). In synthetic versions of testosterone approved only for use on adult males, the risk of blood-clotting is well-known; for teenage girls, drug induced thickened blood is pushing its way round a smaller female cardiovascular system, thinner arteries and smaller veins. The long-term consequences of medical experimentation on children diagnosed as 'transgender' are not known.

"You can't make a child transgender"

What does this matter though, when it's all in service of helping children to become their 'authentic selves'? This treatment helps transgender kids and you can't *make* a child transgender so it's not a problem for anyone else is it? The proliferation of blogs and support forums from a growing community of 'detransitioners' puts the lie to this blithe assertion (Cari, 2016). We hear more and more distressing stories from young people - predominantly but not exclusively young lesbian women - who thought they were 'trans' but on reaching full adult maturity, realise they are not. Young women who stop taking testosterone are left with the irreversible effects of deeper, hoarser voices and increased body hair as well as, in many cases, an irreversible double mastectomy.

It may be impossible to make just any child 'trans' but it is certainly possible to increase persistence in small children who already believe they are the opposite sex. 'Social transition' of pre-pubertal children means nothing less than daily affirmation and reinforcement by trusted adults that a little boy (for example) is really a girl. By the time he reaches puberty he is effectively conditioned and we have created the fear of the 'wrong' puberty which will now, in the child's mind, turn 'her' into a boy. The need for blockers is created. Blockers are promoted by activists as "reversible" and a chance for the child to "buy time to decide" but clearly they work to create persistence, as the point that children typically change their minds is during the natural puberty which blockers prevent. According to the Tavistock clinic, 90% of children on blockers progress to cross-sex hormones; doctors in the US boast a 100% conversion rate (Adams, 2016). Blockers clearly ensure that children do not change their minds. Denied the experience of emerging sexuality in their own biological bodies, these children are left in a state of suspended childhood, stuck in a pre-sexual understanding of who they are; meanwhile the child's peer group surges forward on the path of sexual maturation and leave the gender confused child far behind. The need for cross-sex hormones as early as possible is thus created (Transgender Trend, 2016e).

We have embarked on a re-education programme to teach *all* children that if you are non-conforming, if you don't fit in with your same-sex peers, if you are 'different' in relation to how you feel about being a boy or being a girl, this means you are 'transgender'. We are systematically conditioning all children into a belief in 'gender identity' as the real distinction between boys and girls. We have simultaneously outlawed children's access to facts and information by ensuring that all professionals and trusted adults are giving them the same story. This can only have no effect in *creating* 'transgender kids' if you believe that children do not learn what we teach them.

Conclusion

'Transgender kids' as a definition exists only in a mythical world outside of any wider cultural context. Our children though, are growing up in a specific culture in which there is enormous pressure to fit gender stereotypes; which views children and adolescents as fully autonomous agents making free choices; which glamorises transgender identity; where homophobia and misogyny are still rife and within which, children are being taught 'gender identity' ideology as truth.

'Transgender kids' is not a scientific or medical term but a political one. There has been no scientific breakthrough over the last few years, no globally-trumpeted announcement of the discovery that sexual dimorphism in humans lies in their personal, subjective feelings and not in their male and female biology; no new theory of mind which bestows on children the power to change reality by wishing hard enough. What we have been witnessing is not only a medical experiment on some children's bodies but a psychological experiment on all children's minds. What will happen if we tell teenage girls that their male classmate is now a 'girl' and that the reality that he is male is not true? How will deception and gaslighting of children affect their security and their trust in adults? What will be the cumulative effects of cognitive dissonance on the mental health of children who are no longer allowed to name reality? In trying to protect a minority group we have redefined all boys and girls as 'identities' rather than sexes. There is already plenty of evidence, not least in the confused words of children and adolescents themselves throughout the media, of the devastating impact of this mass societal abuse of young people's trust.

With a non-evidence based medical pathway set in stone and an untested unscientific ideology being promoted as truth from the earliest age, we are witnessing an unprecedented and comprehensive experiment being conducted on the children of this generation. No studies on the long-term effects of the transgender experiment on children have yet been carried out.

References

Adams, T. (2016) Transgender children: the parents and doctors on the frontline, *The Guardian*
https://www.theguardian.com/society/2016/nov/13/transgender-children-the-parents-and-doctors-on-the-frontline?CMP=twt_gu

Allsortsyouth (2014) http://www.allsortsyouth.org.uk/wp-content/uploads/2014/02/Trans-Inclusion-Schools Toolkit.pdf

APA (2007) *Report of the APA Task Force on the Sexualization of Girls*
http://www.apa.org/pi/women/programs/girls/report.aspx

Bailey, M. and Zucker, K. (1995) Childhood Sex-Typed Behavior and Sexual Orientation: A Conceptual Analysis and Quantitative Review. *Developmental Psychology,* Vol 31, No 1. pp 43-55

Banned By Trans – Who's Censoring Who? (undated) *Censored by Transpolitics: A Masterpost*
https://bannedbytrans.wordpress.com/masterpost

BBC (2016*) Analysis Beyond Binary* http://www.bbc.co.uk/programmes

BBC iPM (2016) *"I'm not a boy or a girl. I'm both." A ten-year-old talks about being gender non-binary and explaining to family, friends and teachers that going on living as a girl "just felt wrong".*
http://www.bbc.co.uk/programmes

BBC News (2016) *Gender identity clinic for young people sees referrals double* http://www.bbc.co.uk/news/uk-36010664

BBC Today (2016) http://www.bbc.co.uk/programmes

Blakemore, S., Burnett, S., and Dahil, R. (2010) The Role of Puberty in the Developing Adolescent Brain, *Human Brain Mapping* https://www.ncbi.nlm.nih.gov/pmc/articles/PMC3410522/ doi: 10.1002/hbm.21052

Boghani, P. (2015) *When Transgender Kids Transition, Medical Risks are Both Known and Unknown* http://www.pbs.org/wgbh/frontline/article/when-transgender-kids-transition-medical-risks-are-both-known-and-unknown

Campbell, D. (2016) NHS figures show 'shocking' rise in self-harm among young, *The Guardian* https://www.theguardian.com/society/2016/oct/23/nhs-figures-show-shocking-rise-self-harm-young-people

Cantor, J. (2016) Do trans- kids stay trans- when they grow up? *Sexology Today!* http://www.sexologytoday.org/2016/01/do-trans-kids-stay-trans-when-they-grow_99.html

Cari (2016) *Female detransition and reidentification: Survey results and interpretation* http://guideonragingstars.tumblr.com/post/149877706175/female-detransition-and-reidentification-survey

Channel 4 (2016) *Kids on the Edge* http://www.channel4.com/programmes/kids-on-the-edge/on-demand

Childline (undated) *Support with Transitioning* https://www.childline.org.uk/info-advice/your-feelings/sexual-identity/transgender-identity

Commons Select Committee (2016) *'Widespread' sexual harassment and violence in schools must be tackled* https://www.parliament.uk/business/committees/committees-a-z/commons-select/women-and-equalities-committee/news-parliament-2015/sexual-harassment-and-violence-in-schools-report-published-16-17

Crown Prosecution Service (undated) *Schools Project - homophobic and transphobic bullying and hate crime* http://www.cps.gov.uk/northwest/working_with_you/hate_crime_schools_project/schools_project___lgbt_hate_crime

Davey, M. (2016) More young girls asking GPs about genital cosmetic surgery, study finds, *The Guardian* https://www.theguardian.com/lifeandstyle/2016/oct/06/more-young-girls-asking-gp-genital-cosmetic-surgery-study-finds?

Dearden, L. (2015) *Breast ironing in the UK: Girls' breasts being flattened with hot stones and metal in 'absurdly harmful' tradition* http://www.independent.co.uk/news/uk/home-news/breast-ironing-in-the-uk-girls-breasts-being-flattened-with-hot-stones-and-metal-in-absurdly-harmful-a6693266.html

Donnelly L. (2017) Don't call pregnant women 'expectant mothers' as it might offend transgender people, BMA says *The Telegraph* http://www.telegraph.co.uk/news/2017/01/29/dont-call-pregnant-women-expectant-mothers-might-offend-transgender

Doughty, S. (2016) *Children as young as 13 to be asked whether they are 'gender fluid', 'demi-girl' or 'intersex': Official survey asks pupils to pick from a list of TWENTY-FIVE genders* http://www.dailymail.co.uk/news/article-3420203/Are-gender-fluid-demi-girl-intersex.html

Fine, C. (2013) New insights into gendered brain wiring, or a perfect case study in neurosexism? *The Conversation.* http://theconversation.com/new-insights-into-gendered-brain-wiring-or-a-perfect-case-study-in-neurosexism-21083

Fox, M. (2016) *FDA Steps Up Warnings for Testosterone, Other Steroids* http://www.nbcnews.com/health/health-news/fda-steps-warnings-testosterone-other-steroids-n672681

Gendered Intelligence (2017) *Trans Youth Camping Trip* http://genderedintelligence.co.uk/trans-youth/camping

Gill, J. (2016) BBC defend CBBC's Just a Girl following claim that transgender series is "inappropriate" for young audience. *Radio Times.* http://www.radiotimes.com/news/2016-10-30/bbc-defend-cbbcs-just-a-girl-following-claim-that-transgender-series-is-inappropriate-for-young-audience

GIRES (2017) *Classroom Lesson Plans* http://www.gires.org.uk/education/classroom-lesson-plans

GirlGuiding (undated) https://www.girlguiding.org.uk/about-us/what-makes-guiding-special/our-mission

Hatton, E. and Trautner, M., (2011) Equal Opportunity Objectification? The Sexualization of Men and Women on the Cover of Rolling Stone. *Sexuality & Culture* 15 (3): 256 DOI: 10.1007/s12119-011-9093-2

Hembree, W., Cohen-Kettenis,P., Delemarre-van de Waal, H., Gooren, L. and Meyer, W., Spack, N., Tangpricha, V. and Montori, V. (2009) Endocrine Treatment of Transsexual Persons:An Endocrine Society

Clinical Practice Guideline *The Journal of Clinical Endocrinology & Metabolism*, Volume 94, Issue 9, 1 pp 3132–3154, https://doi.org/10.1210/jc.2009-0345

Jewett, C. (2017) *Women Fear Drug They Used to Halt Puberty Led to Health Problems* http://californiahealthline.org/news/women-fear-drug-they-used-to-halt-puberty-led-to-health-problems

Kirby, J. (2016) *Unhappiness With Their Gender* http://www.independent.co.uk/life-style/health-and-families/health-news/transgender-gender-childline-nspcc-record-numbers-lgbt-trans-rights-a7470856.html

Kleeman, J. (2015) Transgender children: 'This is who he is – I have to respect that' *The Guardian.* https://www.theguardian.com/society/2015/sep/12/transgender-children-have-to-respect-who-he-is

Lyons, K. (2016) Gender Identity Clinic Service Under Strain as Referral Rates *Soar. The Guardian,* 10 July 2016

Miller, S., Booth Church, E. and Poole, C. (2017) Ages & Stages: How Children Use Magical Thinking, *Early Childhood Today* https://www.scholastic.com/teachers/articles/teaching-content/ages-stages-how-children-use-magical-thinking

Mirror.co.uk (2011) *Children of 12 to be allowed gender drugs to prepare for sex change* http://www.mirror.co.uk/news/technology-science/children-of-12-to-be-allowed-gender-drugs-121674

National Centre for Transgender Terminology (2104) *Transgender Terminology* http://www.transequality.org/issues/resources/transgender-terminology

Peck, S. (2015) 250 children's toy adverts on British TV analysed - it's worse than we thought. *The Telegraph.* http://www.telegraph.co.uk/women/family/250-childrens-toy-adverts-on-british-tv-analysed-its-worse-than/

Peitzmeier, S., Gardner, I., Weinand, J., Corbet, A. and Acevedo, K. (2107) Sexuality Health impact of chest binding among transgender adults: a community-engaged, cross-sectional study, *Journal Culture, Health* Volume 19

Papadopoulis, L. (2010) *Sexualisation of Young People* http://drlinda.co.uk/sexualisation-of-young-people

Sanchez Manning (2015) *Children as young as FOUR being given transgender lessons which encourage them to explore their 'gender identities'* http://www.dailymail.co.uk/news/article-3298715/Children-young-FOUR-given-transgender-lessons-encourage-explore-gender-identities.html#ixzz4pWP1MlB0

Sandman, G. (2016) *Struggling to Breathe: Councils tell schools to give transgender pupils 'extra PE breaks' because of chest-binding practice* https://www.thesun.co.uk/news/1527158/councils-tell-schools-to-give-transgender-pupils-extra-pe-breaks-because-of-chest-binding-practice

Scutti, S. (2013) *Transgender Youth: Are Puberty-Blocking Drugs An Appropriate Medical Intervention?* http://www.medicaldaily.com/transgender-youth-are-puberty-blocking-drugs-appropriate-medical-intervention-247082

Spillet, R. (2015) *Children as young as three should be taught about transgender issues using story books about PENGUINS, MPs told* http://www.dailymail.co.uk/news/article-3243313/Children-young-three-taught-transgender-issues-MPs-told.html#ixzz4pWQ1LdGI

Sweet, E. (2015) Toys Are More Divided by Gender Now Than They Were 50 Years Ago. *The Atlantic.* https://www.theatlantic.com/business/archive/2014/12/toys-are-more-divided-by-gender-now-than-they-were-50-years-ago/383556

Taylor, D. (2015) Children seeking gender identity advice sees 100% increase, says NHS, *The Guardian.* https://www.theguardian.com/society/2015/nov/05/children-seeking-gender-identity-advice-sees-100-increase-nhs?

Theroux, L. (2015) *Transgender Kids*. BBC2 http://www.bbc.co.uk/programmes

Topping, A. (2017) Campaigners hail school decision to let pupils choose gender identity *The Guardian* //www.theguardian.com/world/2017/feb/19/st-pauls-girls-school-pupils-choose-gender-indentity?

Transgender Reality (2016) *"Do you feel uncomfortable with yourself in some way?"* https://transgenderreality.com/2016/07/30/do-you-feel-uncomfortable-with-yourself-in-some-way

Transgender Trend (2016) *Transgender Diagnosis and Treatment of Kids Is Not Up For Debate* http://www.TransgenderTrend.com/trans gender-diagnosis-and-treatment-of-kids-is-not-up-for-debate

—. (2016a) *UK CBBC Children's TV: I Am Leo* http://www.Transgender Trend.com/uk-cbbc-childrens-tv-i-am-leo

—. (2016b) *Teaching Transgender Doctrine in Schools – "A Bizarre Educational Experiment"* https://www.TransgenderTrend.com/teaching-transgender-doctrine-in-schools-a-bizarre-educational-experiment

—. (2016c) *Woman's Hour on Teenage Girls At Tavistock Clinic* http://www.Transgender Trend.com/womans-hour-on-teenage-girls-at-tavistock-clinic

—. (2016d) *Speech Language Assessment, Autism and Transition*
https://www.Transgender Trend.com/tag/tavistock-clinic

—. (2016e) *UK Doctor Prescribes Cross-Sex Hormones to Twelve-Year-Old*
http://www.TransgenderTrend.com/uk-doctor-prescribes-cross-sex-hormones-twelve-year-old

Wadsworth, J. (2106) *Brighton and Hove News*
http://www.brightonandhovenews.org/2016/04/19/brighton-and-hove-schools-ask-three-year-olds-what-gender-if-any-they-identify-with

4thWaveNow (2016) *Tumblr Snags Another Girl, but her therapist-mom knows a thing or two about social contagion*
https://4thwavenow.com/2016/02/29/tumblr-snags-another-girl-but-her-therapist-mom-knows-a-thing-or-two-about-social-contagion

CHAPTER THREE

GENDERED MIS-INTELLIGENCE: THE FABRICATION OF 'THE TRANSGENDER CHILD'

HEATHER BRUNSKELL-EVANS

Twenty years ago, the 'transgender child' would not have made sense to the general public, nor would it have made sense to young people. Today, children and adolescents declare themselves transgender, the NHS diagnoses 'gender dysphoria', and laws and policy are invented which uphold young people's 'choice' to transition and to authorize the stages at which medical intervention is permissible and desirable.

The current narrative of 'the transgender child' has numerous, attendant strands: although previously unrecognized, children born into the 'wrong' body are alleged to have always existed; parents are 'brave' when they accept their son is 'really' a girl (and vice versa); listening to the child's experiences of gender non-conformity helps revolutionizes hidebound, sexist and outdated ideas about gender; and medical intervention and legal recognition of 'the transgender child' is a sign of a tolerant, liberal and humane society. What is the provenance of such a narrative? On what scientific medical, psychological or philosophical basis is the 'truth' founded?

I argue that 'the transgender child' is not natural but a newly constructed category of person forged out of official knowledges, the play of power politics, and misdirected liberal values. These combined relations of knowledge-power-ethics (Foucault, 1982) construct the composite picture of 'the transgender child' that we recognize today in the UK in broadcast and social media. I demonstrate that the figure of 'the transgender child' is no more objective and no less political than the figure of 'the pathological homosexual', 'the macho-man' and 'the inferior woman' that conventional liberal wisdom is now happy to consign to history. I suggest that 'the transgender child' should be equally understood as a socially constructed identity that should be rejected. In contrast to enabling freedom, by insisting gender is inherent rather than a social construct, the gendered intelligence offered by transgender doctrine to children, parents and society at large endorses the very gendered norms of 'masculinity' and 'femininity' it is purported to revolutionize. In contrast to the idea that transgendering a young person is progressive and humane I argue it is politically reactionary and an egregious abrogation by society of responsibility to protect children from harm.

Liberal Wisdom

A small event serves to illustrate the ubiquity of the current liberal wisdom that 'the transgender child' is 'real' and that transgendering children is progressive. A young woman in her early twenties does odd jobs for me in the garden now and again. She is fascinated by the fact that I am an academic who analyzes sex, gender and sexuality, but at the same time I am skeptical about current knowledges and politics of transgendering children.

One day, during moments when I took her cups of tea and chatted, she questioned me about my critical views. She informed me that in ancient times the 'shamans' revered sex-indeterminate individuals as nearer to gods than other mortals. In the present day, men dressing as women is an expression of their 'feminine side', thus demonstrating that feminine men have existed throughout time. I assured her that I can really understand her spiritual perspective on the issue of gender indeterminacy. It seems to me that freezing 'masculinity' as biologically inherent is restrictive of the range of human expressions open to men (and women). I quipped, truthfully, that I rather like men in dresses and find men who are *uncomfortable* with 'masculinity' far more attractive at every level of human connection than their less self-reflexive peers. She was perplexed by what she judged to be my contradictory perspective – my appreciation of gender fluidity and yet my avowed critical analysis of the theory and practice of transgendering children. Each of my replies was unsatisfactory to her, but rather than deterring, they provoked further questions. Surely, she probed, to be opposed to transgendering children is tantamount to resurrecting 'the patriarchy'?

The moment my friend's moral assessment was out of her mouth, I knew I had fallen into the (by now) familiar 'rabbit hole' when casual discussion about transgenderism occurs. A dichotomy is erected, blocking any other view or thoughtful exploration: progressive people are supportive of transgendering children; critics are transphobes who fear a breakdown of traditional gender roles. Experience has taught me that once ethics are framed in this way – a direction of travel usually arrived at with great speed and in this instance about four minutes – there is no gainsaying my interlocutor's belief in her own alleged moral high-ground. In contrast, I become immediately aligned with bigotry and transphobia.

What I would have liked to have replied on this occasion is that whilst I share my friend's aspiration for gender freedom we have a moral obligation, particularly with regard to children and adolescents, to open transgender doctrine to critical scrutiny. To truly defend progressivism, we would need to examine the following: Are the sex-indeterminate men of 'ancient times' identical with 21st century transwomen? What relation does transgender doctrine propose exists between biological sex and gender? What kinds of persons do transgender adults assert 'transgender children' *are*? What exactly are the medical and legal changes lobbied for by transgender activists? What are the long-term consequences for children of social and/or medical transition? Do the doctors and the lobbyists fulfil their shared declared aim of releasing children from gender oppression, and if not, why not?

The Making of 'The Transgender Adult'

In order to reflect upon ethics and whether any particular subjective identity is freeing or constraining, it is necessary to first understand how the identity was configured or 'put together' (Foucault, 1994). In order to examine the component parts that make up the narrative of 'the transgender child' as a real, ahistorical, naturally occurring figure it is important to briefly explore the figure of 'the transgender adult' since 'the transgender child' is its off-shoot (Jeffreys, 2014).

Transgender adults repeatedly claim that their gender was not aligned with their 'assigned' sex at birth. The concept of assigned suggests that when babies are born an evaluative judgement is made, one that can *misrecognize* the sex of the child (Jensen, 2017). However, the phrase 'assigned' is only relevant to intersex people, about 0.05% of the population, whose genitalia at birth are ambiguous (or approximately 1.7% if the percentage includes later discovery for example of intersex chromosome composition, gonadal structure, hormone levels, and/or the structure of the internal genital duct systems). The fact that a tiny percentage of people are born intersex – the category of person referred to by my friend – does not negate the fact that the overwhelming majority of people are born with unambiguous genitalia, including those children medically designated as transgender. With very little exception babies occupy a sex-category, male or female, based on objective, observed reality. Since male and female are discernible biological categories what does it mean for someone unambiguously female or male to claim she is in fact male (or vice versa) (Jensen, 2017)? What is the political and social context out of which such a claim, bizarre to the ears of the general public 30 years ago, apparently now makes sense?

The claim that one's gender is inherent but that biology can be socially constructed has emerged out the complex history of LGBTQ knowledges and politics. In the 1970s and 1980s a paradigm shift in thought about sex and gender occurred which drove a wedge between biological sex (the division between male and female based on reproductive capacity) and social gender ('masculinity' and 'femininity'). Lesbian and gay theorists/activists utilized these new ideas to critique the medical designation of heterosexual men and women as psychologically healthy whilst homosexuals were designated deviant. They demonstrate that that the figure of 'the pathological homosexual' was not an objective naturally occurring type of person but a socially constructed identity brought into being by medicine and then reified as if natural (Weeks, 1985; Mort,1987). In other words, gender and sexuality have a political history, with which medicine was complicit and helped reproduce.

The LGB community began to refuse to see themselves as defective, disordered heterosexuals and to openly transgress gender stereotypes in order to shine a light on the gender myths of medicine and wider society (Murray, 2017). During the 1990s, queer theory was developed which built upon the lesbian and gay examination of the socially constructed nature of gender, sexual acts and identities and it developed a theory of gender non-binarism. Queer politics very quickly became less about the original gay movement's analysis of sex and gender and structures of oppression, and more about the rights of gay people to play with and transgress gender norms (Jeffreys, 2014).

A small transgender movement had sprung up alongside the LGB movement in the 1970s and 1980s, and although connected, nevertheless transgender adults retained different aims, aspirations and politics (Jeffreys, 2014). During this period, although the number of individuals claiming to be transgender was minimal, numbers began to grow in line with the exponential growth of medical technologies – hormone treatment, breast implants and the construction of artificial vaginas and so on – that attempted to convert anatomical sex (Raymond, 1979). By the 1990s, partly because of the potential for networking created by the Internet, the transgender movement finally became firmly established. It began to make the following claims overturning the insights of the sex/gender distinction:

gender is not socially constructed but inherent; the biological division of human beings into two sexed categories is socially constructed; it is possible to be born into the 'wrong' body; medical 'gender' transition is a human right; transgender people are marginalized and oppressed by the same hetero-sexism that had discriminated against lesbian and gay people; transgenderism is sexually transgressive and thus politically progressive (Jeffreys, 2014). Considerable social, political and legal changes have occurred in response to transgender lobbying, and there is increasing acquiescence by governments, medicine, and the law to demands for transgender rights (Jeffreys, 2014).

By the 21st century, the idea that transgender people belong to an oppressed category and that their suffering needs to be alleviated through medical intervention, has become firmly established as incontrovertible. The American Psychological Association, for example, currently describes transgender and gender nonconforming (TGNC) people as those who have a gender identity that is "not fully aligned with their assigned sex at birth" (2015: 832). The organization stipulates that in the last 20 years, there has been an "increase in knowledge informed by the TGNC community which has resulted in the development of progressively more trans-affirmative practice across the multiple health disciplines" (2015: 832). The data suggests "extensive experiences of stigma and discrimination reported by TGNC people […] including increased rates of depression and suicidality" (2015: 832). It has produced guidelines which "assist psychologists in the provision of culturally competent, developmentally appropriate, and trans-affirmative psychological practice […] supportive of the identities and life experiences of TGNC people" (2015: 832-833).

In conclusion, the current transgender movement gives the appearance of progressivism but has returned to a traditional naturalization of femininity and masculinity. The common liberal wisdom that transgendering young people is progressive emerges out of the success of the transgender movement in persuading that queering gender for adults is both progressive and revolutionary. The current transgender movement is not an extension of the past efforts of the lesbian and gay rights movement to deconstruct sexist and hetero-sexist myths and stereo-types (Murray, 2017). In reifying gender, transgenderism gives credence to the very gender myths that lesbian and gay activists originally spurned (Murray, 2017). The philosopher Terri Murray argues the transgender movement is not a natural sequel to feminist and gay liberation united in opposing heterosexist mythology, rather it:

"... divides and conquers the once-powerful counter-cultural movement, hijacking its language and mimicking its political posture to disguise its opposite intent" (Murray 2017: 6).

Transgender individuals who have led the transgender movement are well-positioned establishment figures who have the full backing of the media in promoting their cause (Murray, 2017). Gender as a social construction, "once wielded by the liberal left against conservative sexist and heterosexist social norms" has now been "retooled as a weapon in the armory of a regressive politics that is not only sexist but homophobic" (Murray, 2017: 6, 7). "Today's transgender movement reinforces the myth that 'men' and 'women' are different species of human being, not just reproductively, but mentally – with different desires, different needs, different aptitudes, and different minds" (Murray, 2017: 7).

How is this reactionary move played out on and through the bodies of children?

Medicine: The 'Making' of 'The Transgender Child'

During the same period that transgender movement was gathering political traction for the reality of 'the transgender adult', 'the transgender child' was beginning to make its appearance. During the 1990s, trans led organizations such as Gender Identity Research and Education Society (GIRES) (GIRES, 2017) and Mermaids (Mermaids, 2017) spearheaded demand for early social/ medical intervention on the grounds gender nonconforming or gender defiant children would grow up to be transgender adults. Re-assignment of gender in childhood would spare individuals the future trauma of reaching adulthood in 'the wrong body'.

A collaborative symposium took place in 2005 between GIRES, Mermaids, and an international collection of doctors and medical researchers (Department of Health, 2008). The Department of Health discloses that since this time "GIRES and Mermaids remain in close contact with these medical professionals" (Department of Health, 2008: 3). The symposium achieved a major success for the transgender lobby with the publication by The Endocrine Society in 2009 of new clinical practice guidelines for endocrine treatment of transgender youth (Endocrine Society, 2009). The advice has not been without controversy, but nevertheless it has been adopted, as we shall see shortly, by the most specialized gender identity clinic for children in the UK, the Gender Identity Development Service (GIDS).

A further outcome of the international collaboration was the publication in the UK of NHS guidelines for advising "gender variant children and young adults and their families" (Department of Health, 2008:3). Parents are informed that transgenderism results from a mismatch between "the sex" to which their children were "assigned at birth" and the child's "inner sense of knowing" they are boys or girls (Department of Health, 2008: 4). For some individuals, "the way they look on the outside does not fit how they feel inside" (Department of Health, 2008: 4). Gender variance in children can show itself in "the way they behave, in their dress or play" (Department of Health, 2008: 4). The genitalia of a child and the brain can have "distinctly different male and female characteristics" (Department of Health, 2008: 4). Some babies can be predisposed to a future mismatch between "gender identity and sex appearance" (Department of Health, 2008: 5). "Gender identity appears to be indelible from birth" (Department of Health, 2008: 13).

The NHS guidelines urge parents to accept their children's 'real' gender as the most appropriate and loving response to what is a physical condition. They assure parents that through psychological and medical support the child's sex appearance can be aligned with their true gender, and thus the child's anxiety about living in a society where other people's appearance and gender 'match' will be minimized. The earlier their child's gender variance is addressed "the more comfortable and happy your child may be as an adult" (Department of Health, 2008:11). The publication offers numerous website resources for parents and children, including those of GIRES, Mermaids, Gendered Intelligence, and a Department of Health Website.

In conclusion, parents are left in no doubt that their children's gender non-compliance arises out of their child's body. The most loving response of any parent, without any other framework of understanding, is to support the child to transition. How could any parent, without access to alternative ways of understanding, refuse the therapies offered or dispute this medical assessment of their child as a medically verifiable?

Neuro-sexism: Female and Male Brains

The idea of the sexed brain disseminated by the NHS to parents as objective truth is unproven (Eliot, 2010; Fine, 2010, 2017; Fine et al 2013; Joel et al, 2015; Joel 2016). Daphna Joel, Professor of Neuroscience, informs that although the genitals are unmistakably dimorphic the brain is not: brains belong to a single heterogeneous category rather than two distinct categories (Joel et al, 2015). From conception to puberty children have multiple and continuous gendered experiences which, because of the brain's plasticity, can leave slight neurological traces. Lise Eliot (2010), also a Professor of Neuroscience, says infant brains are so malleable that any small differences become amplified over time, as parents, teachers, peers – and the culture at large – unwittingly reinforce gender stereotypes. Children themselves exacerbate the differences by reproducing the behavioural patterns expected and rewarded by their care-givers (Eliot, 2010).

Cordelia Fine (Fine et al 2013), Professor of Cognitive Psychology, argues that those neuroscientists who claim that brains are sexed offer untested stereo-types based on speculation (Fine et al 2013). By failing to look at social influences on small brain difference, research is subtly "neuro-sexist", reinforcing and legitimizing gender stereotypes in ways that are not scientifically justified (Fine et al 2013). Instead of recognizing that new developments of neuroscience open up important opportunities to challenge social assumptions through rigorous, reflective scientific inquiry and debate, scientists sometimes contribute to inaccurate and harmful lay misunderstandings of what neuroscience tells us (Fine et al 2013). The suggestion there is a 'boy brain' and 'girl brain' makes us overlook the important point that boys' and girls' behaviours are far more similar than they are different (2010, 2017). Psychological research provides extremely strong evidence for behavioural similarities between the sexes, and provides no evidence that modest behavioural differences are associated with brain difference rather than culture (Fine 2010, 2017).

Given that there is no hard-scientific evidence that demonstrates, for example, that a biologically male individual possesses a distinctly male brain, it is even more indemonstrable that a biologically male individual could possess a distinctly female brain. Nevertheless, the number of children and teenagers now diagnosed with gender dysphoria, the etiology of which is traced to the brain, is increasing year upon year in the UK. Since the belief in the syndrome of 'the transgender child' is growing, the first port of call for young people and their parents is the GP. GIRES has designed an e-learning course as a resource for GPs to help them "respond to the needs of adults and young people experiencing gender dysphoria" (Royal College of General Practitioners, 2017). The purpose of such a resource, GIRES argues, is because GPs have a crucial role in providing appropriate medical care for trans people, including those who are non-binary or non-gender, and service providers must be aware that children who do not receive prompt support for their gender variance are at risk of committing suicide (GIRES, 2017). GPs refer parents and children to gender identity clinics, in particular to GIDS, first established for adults in 1989 by the Tavistock and Portman NHS Foundation Trust in London.

Treatment at GIDS is developed in three sequential stages. Firstly, before puberty, the clinic works with the family and school to provide psychological support for children "exhibiting cross-gender behaviour or dress" (Department of Health, 2008: 16). Secondly, since 2011 and the advice of The Endocrine Society described above, hormone blocking medication can be administered in the early teenage years. Since there is no "physical test … for detecting gender variance that may develop into adult dysphoria … clinicians must rely on the young person's own account" (Department of Health, 2008: 17). Thirdly, if the young person makes a firm decision to remain permanently in the new gender role, cross-sex hormonal medication can be offered after the age of 16. Parents are warned that some of the physical changes induced by cross-sex hormone medication, including infertility, are difficult or even impossible to reverse. Young people are not eligible for surgery to alter the body to conform as nearly as possible to their gender identity – such as removal of the testes, penis, ovaries and breasts – until they have reached the age of eighteen years (Department of Health, 2008).

When pressed for a cause for soaring figures Polly Carmichael, consultant clinical psychologist and the director of GIDS, admits no single explanation can be found but proffers an answer based on societal change rather than science: transgenderism is now socially acceptable; we are increasingly aware of "gender diverse people"; transgender organizations have disseminated greater awareness to parents, children and others and how to access clinics; and "an increased awareness of the possibilities around physical treatments for younger adolescents" (Tavistock Announcement, 2017).

In conclusion, the knowledge and the services provided for children by the NHS are based on little other than gender stereotypes, dependence on the young person's personal sense of identity, and speculative unproven brain science. Medicine *assumes* what it needs to prove, and as such it is has become caught up in a circular form of argumentation. By pre-supposing gender *a priori*, the concept of non-binary gender, does not allow for an escape from gender. The medical advice pre-supposes gender *a priori,* so that when individuals do not conform to gender stereo-types this 'evidence' is not taken as a flaw in the concept that gender is natural and intrinsic, but rather as its proof (Murray, 2016). The seemingly compassionate 'progressive' clinical response reinforces the very binary from which the person is allegedly freed (Murray, 2016).

Counter-discourses are now springing up which dare to challenge the wisdom of medical advice and its impact on young people and their parents. Transgender Trend, an international group of concerned parents, points to the absence of public scrutiny of the exponential rise in the number of children referred to GIDS (Transgender Trend, 2017) (see Davies-Arai, Chapter Two this volume). The group asserts it should cause serious public concern that practices of transgendering children involve the use of puberty suppression, cross-sex hormonal medication that harms children's reproductive capacity, their bodily integrity and future physical and psychological health, and possible surgery involving the amputation of penises and breasts that cannot be re-attached (Transgender Trend, 2016). Setting children on a path of medicalization with irreversible life-long effects is an unprecedented experiment with which the whole of society has become complicit (Transgender Trend, 2017a). Moreover, the claim that without medical treatment young people will be driven to thoughts of suicide is based on flawed methodology and manipulative statistical analysis (Transgender Trend, 2017).

Transgender Trend urges extreme caution before treating children since the alleged 'fact' promulgated by transgender adults and now medical professionals that gender identity is inherent and can override external sex-characteristics in determining whether one is male or female is completely untested. Its application to children, who are in the process of physically maturing and developing their identities, contradicts all other established knowledges of child development and psychology (Transgender Trend, 2015). None of us is privileged with foresight to know what the long-term consequences will be on a girl, for example, who is currently supported in her belief she is 'really' a boy, and helped by her adult caregivers to transition from 'boyhood' to 'manhood'. She may grow up to realize that she can never, however many hormones she has ingested or however many surgical operations she has undergone, truly achieve the body of a man with its capacity for reproduction and sexual pleasure. The idea that you can actually be a boy trapped in a girl's body' or vice versa is not backed by credible brain science, and the medical treatment pathway is not backed by long-term research or any evidence base about safety or harm (Transgender Trend, 2015).

'Gendered Intelligence': The 'Making' of 'The Transgender Child'

In association with GIRES and Mermaids, Gendered Intelligence helps construct 'the transgender child'. Established in 2008, it holds an increasingly prominent position as a provider of advice to educational institutions and to other advisory bodies (Gendered Intelligence, 2017). It conveys alleged 'truths' of gender non-binarism to children in schools in England and Wales through workshops and assemblies at Key Stages 1-2 (ages six to eleven) and Key Stages 3-4 (ages eleven to sixteen). The people who operationalize the workshops and advice have received a two-day in-house course which trains practicing transgender psychotherapists, therapists and counsellors who are transgender to become the "experts" or "gender identity specialists" (Gendered Intelligence Training, 2017).

Gendered Intelligence makes its political aspirations overt. These are to: increase the visibility of young trans people's lives and raise awareness of their needs, across the UK and beyond; help create community cohesion across the whole of the trans community and the wider LGBT community throughout the UK; and improve public understanding of the diversity and complexity of gender through lobbying and consultation on public bodies (Gendered Intelligence, 2017).

Jay Stewart, co-founder and CEO of Gendered Intelligence, tells that he was "assigned female at birth" but now "lives as a man" (Stewart, 2015). He is an academic who is theoretically grounded in queer theory and his ideas about gender non-binarism comprise the epistemic and political foundations of the organization (Stewart, 2015, 2017). As well as queer theory, he argues the philosophy of existentialism is extremely important because it helps describe the capacity of human beings to transcend the gender binary through willful acts of 'self-choosing'. Stewart says three philosophers of existentialism have been personally empowering to him. The first is Simone de Beauvoir, a 20th century philosopher who argues "One is not born but becomes a woman"; the second is Fredric Nietzsche, a 19th century philosopher, who argues "There is no doer behind the doing"; and the third is Judith Butler, an eminent 21st century queer theorist, who argues "There is no gender identity behind the expression of gender" (Stewart, 2015). I shall focus here on Butler (1990, 2004) and de Beauvoir (1949).

Children's Existential 'Choice'

Butler argues the sexed body (i.e. being male or female) is gendered from birth by culture, and then reproduced by us through our 'doing' (Butler, 1990). Since binary gender is forged through performative action, she proposes that *adult* subversion of binary gender can occur by queering it, namely playing with gender expression and presentation in a range of ways that challenge and undermine its normativity. In Butler's view transgenderism "should be a matter of choice, an exercise of freedom" (2004: 88). To choose one's gender is about "the ability to live and breathe and move and would no doubt belong somewhere in what is called a philosophy of freedom" (2004: 88).

Stewart applies Butler's philosophy of adult self-choice to transgress gender norms to children and teenagers. Echoing Butler's proposition that the transgenderism is a philosophy of freedom, he insists that for young people, and the adults who support them: "Now is the time to come together ... and get behind the right to express ourselves, get behind Gendered Intelligence and other organizations like us" (Stewart, 2017). The collective aims are the social justice for children and adolescents to be able:

> "To breathe and to move more freely – that is what trans, gender diverse and gender questioning people need – to breathe, to expand our lungs, our bodies, our-selves – let us feel what's right, let us do what's right – right now" (Stewart, 2017).

In order to support his claim that non-binary gender is embedded in the 'self' and can be self-directed by children, Stewart tells that he is informed by Simone de Beauvoir who famously argues in her book *The Second Sex: Facts and Myths*: "One is not born but becomes a woman". Stewart clearly has not grasped de Beauvoir's central thesis about existentialism. She does not propose that becoming a woman is a matter of girls' self-choosing, still less a matter of the self-choosing of boys and men. Her existentialist philosophy of freedom recommends that women *resist* 'becoming a woman' since becoming a woman involves girls and women in internalizing oppressive gender norms. Her overarching point is that in patriarchal cultures, the inequalities between men and women have historically been attributed to 'natural' inequalities arising from male and female biology. Binary sex (which has no intrinsic meaning) is turned into binary gender, a political, externally imposed hierarchy, with two classes, occupying two value positions: male over female, Man over Woman, 'masculinity' over 'femininity'. Whilst binary gender constrains the flourishing, and self-expression of both men and women, girls and women experience by far the most egregious psychological and physical injuries.

Stewart piggy backs upon de Beauvoir's distinction between sex and gender whilst completely inverting her 'facts and myths'. He defines biological essentialism as the idea there is something unalterable about the biological division male or female (Stewart, 2015). In doing so, he untethers gender from its social context, and far from rejecting biological essentialism, he endorses it, mirroring almost exactly the traditional patriarchal claim that gender – namely 'masculinity' and 'femininity' – is pre-social and interior.

In Stewart's view, the "trans, gender diverse and gender questioning" young people he wants his organization to help free are not oppressed by gender in de Beauvoir's sense i.e. gender as structure that mobilizes social inequality between the sexes, or inequality between those with different sexual orientations, or a framework which limits boys' and girls' free expression of which clothes to wear, which toys to play with, and which careers to aspire. In this latter understanding, the obvious solution for liberation and social justice would be to campaign for the abolition of gender! Stewart, in contrast, argues that young people are not oppressed by gender *per se*, but by the current social unacceptability of the 'fact' that there are more than two!

Queering the Child

Soon, Stewart predicts, the theory of non-binary gender will replace the old idea of two distinct gender categories based on genitalia (Stewart, 2017). The old idea of two distinct genders "is (or will be) no longer tenable" […] Gender is more complex, nuanced, political and interesting than that" (Stewart, 2017). Conflating sex with gender, he proposes that the politics of gender reside in the practice of sexing a child at birth based on visual, physical signs – on genitalia to be precise – and on no more, and as such adults can mistake the true 'gender identity' of the child. He argues that reducing people to the sex they are assigned at birth limits the possibilities of human expression to their genitalia. He asks: "Why does the gender binary continue"? It is "absurd, oppressive and dangerous" (Stewart, 2015). The theory of non-binary gender constitutes a paradigm shift not only in knowledge but in politics, and like other paradigm shifts, it is "a revolution, rather than a gentle evolution" (Stewart, 2017). He proclaims: "It looks like that revolution has started" (Stewart, 2017).

Stewart (2017) insists "transgender children are real" as if he anticipates a suggestion that they are a new socially constructed category of person, or perhaps to endorse his proposition that transgenderism has existed across time. He insists that it is young people's *experiences* of gender, now finally listened to and acknowledged, that demonstrates the theory of non-binary gender is objective. Until the success of trans campaigning most scientists – medics, psychologists, sexologists – have been resistant to 'hearing' or 'seeing' the experiences of children (and others) which contradicted their theory of binary gender. He does not acknowledge that at a time when young people are vulnerable because of the teenage search for individuation, identity, and meaning, Gendered Intelligence provides the lens through which young people refract their turmoil and provides a framework for them to make sense. Perhaps it is the predominant, hegemonic voice of transgender adult that is heard by doctors and medics nowadays, and not that of the child.

So, how does Stewart define the needs of the 'real' trans and non-binary children and teenagers whose capacity for existential self-realization he asserts is bringing about a revolution in thought and on behalf of whose freedom Gendered Intelligence campaigns? A specific web platform – *Knowledge is Power: Kapow!* – on the Gendered Intelligence website provides a virtual social space for children and adolescents where ideas of non-binary gender and existential self-choosing are put into a format that children can allegedly understand and make their own. Young people, allegedly 'non-binary' before their immersion in Gendered Intelligence can find information that "offers meaning" and which enables them "to be empowered". This information covers a full range of archived pages linked to resources to help children transition and feel comfortable with transitioning. These include: medical and legal information; links to GIRES and Mermaid; details of on-line fora where children's experiences can be shared and solidarity formed; invitations from Gendered Intelligence to holiday camps for transgender youth; information on where to buy transitional clothing/equipment such as breast binders for girls and genital packers for her trousers so she can appear to have male genitals; and advice on how to navigate alternatives nouns, adjectives and pronouns that cover the whole range of gender as a spectrum (e.g. genderqueer, gender-fluid, agender etc.). "Names, nicknames, pronouns and the language used to describe your body – anything that refers to you is your own choice". The site promises this knowledge not only enriches the lives of children "it's also about changing ourselves and the world for the better! Sharing our own knowledge with others is about ensuring that knowledge circulates and benefits the whole of society" (site).

One of the knowledge resources Gendered Intelligence provides is *The Trans Youth Sexual Health Booklet* (site). The declared aim is to help teenagers and their sexual partners understand the range of experiences they can share as non-binary individuals. A cartoon drawing illustrates the various possibilities. One illustration is of a male body – broad shoulders, beard and body hair – but no penis. Another illustration is of a female body – wide hips, breasts, no body hair – with the addition of a reconstructed, prosthetic penis. It is explained that body modification can be achieved through hormones and surgery, although some trans people do not wish to undergo these interventions. Teenagers are assured this is not a problem, since retaining their biological sex is not an impediment to transitioning. Young people can decide whether they want the "inside" and the "outside" to match, or they can accept the body as it is.

Adolescents are assured that in contrast to traditional sex education in schools which focuses on bodies, "within the trans community we realize that it is identity that's more important" (Gendered Intelligence, 2017). The approach of Gendered Intelligence is that two people with female bodies who identify as male and have sex are "still having gay sex regardless of their bodies because that is how they identify" (Gendered Intelligence, 2017):

> "The fundamental thing ... is that your identity is paramount. A woman is still a woman, even if she enjoys getting blow jobs. A man is still a man, even if he likes getting penetrated vaginally" (Gendered Intelligence, 2017).

Stewart clearly endorses medical technologies that aid sex-transition. However, the main ethos of Gendered Intelligence, and what distinguishes it from other trans-led organizations, is its particular focus on queer theory and the concept of non-binary gender.
The journalist Meaghan Murphy (2017) proposes that melding queer with LGBT, and assuming that LGBTQ comprise an homogenous group, goes some way to explaining why today our "queerest generation" is not progressive on the issue of children and women's liberation. Indeed, the word "queer" is rendered meaningless since it now means any identity one chooses to 'pick and mix', as demonstrated by the array of possibilities that Gendered Intelligence offers young people. Fighting structures of oppression can't happen within an individualist framework, and with endless genders to choose from, the queer movement remains steadfastly misogynistic (Murphy, 2017). The path to revolution, if that is what is desired – and Stewart claims that this is what his organization aspires to – cannot be achieved through boys and men wearing dresses and lip gloss. Jen Izaakson (2017) (see Chapter Eleven, this volume) points out that instead of scrutinizing 'masculinity' and 'femininity' as the products of unequal system of power but by focusing instead on gender performance, gender queer discourse simply opens the door for all the social problems associated with traditional masculinity (e.g. misogyny) and allows patriarchy "easy access to the party" (Izaakson, 2017).

Gendered Mis-Intelligence

Rebecca Reilley-Cooper, a political philosopher, points out there are numerous intellectual inconsistencies with the narrative gender is non-binary that medical and other knowledges simply don't scrutinize or challenge (Reilley-Cooper 2016:3). Firstly, the theory proposes only a proportion of individuals are non-binary, and that the clear majority of people are 'cisgender' i.e. people whose biological body and gender 'fit' (Reilley-Cooper, 2016). Since the majority of people are described as 'cis', Reilley-Cooper points out a new false binary is created between those individuals whose gender fits the heterosexual norm, and those whose identity does not. However, if gender is a spectrum as Gendered Intelligence insists, then everyone is non-binary, since none of us (girls, boys, women, or men) inhabits its furthest points i.e. pure 'masculinity' or pure 'femininity'. If we recognize that we are all non-binary, and that we all to greater or lesser degrees negotiate with gender throughout our lives, we are forced to concede that nobody is deep down 'cisgender' (Reilley-Cooper, 2016).

Secondly, transgender doctrine permits a handful of individuals to opt out of the spectrum altogether by declaring themselves 'agender'. Reilly-Cooper points out that we cannot all be 'agender' for the same reasons we cannot all call ourselves non-binary: 'agender' can only be defined against gender. No explanation is proffered as to why 'agender' individuals can refuse to define themselves in gendered terms whilst others – for example allegedly 'cisgender' people – cannot (Reilly-Cooper, 2016). Thirdly, once we assert that the problem with gender is that we currently recognize only two of them, the obvious question to ask is: how many genders would we have to recognize in order not to be oppressive? The only consistent answer to this is billions, or however many people there are currently living on the planet. Since this is so, "it's not clear how it makes sense or adds anything to our understanding to call any of this stuff 'gender'" (Reilley-Cooper, 2016:4). If we apply this to all the children accessing the Gendered Intelligence website, or to whom Gendered Intelligence talks in schools or on their holiday camps we can ask the following question: "What meaning does the word 'gender' have here, that the word 'personality' cannot capture"? (Reilley-Cooper, 2016:4).

The crucial philosophical tension at the heart the concept of non-binary gender can only be resolved, Reilley-Cooper argues, by rejecting its key tenets. Not only is gender rendered meaningless by the proliferation of genders and their continual expansion, the concept fails in the alleged project of setting young people free from gender. By arguing gender is non-binary and on a spectrum, Stewart merely confirms that gender is innate, and the freedom Gendered Intelligence offers to young people is little other than the search for identity within gender confines. In reconceiving gender as a spectrum not a binary, Stewart does not solve the politics of binary gender but contributes to its de-politicization and naturalization with seriously concerning implications for children.

The Law: The Making of 'The Transgender Child'

Stewart (2015) argues that the legal designation of gender based on genitalia is "an absurd proposition". He insists compliance with gender justice dictates that the law and the human rights of trans persons should not be based on hormonal or surgical reassignment, if this is not the individual's choice, but on his or her existential will to transition, "on the idea of pursuing that which we wish to become" (Stewart, 2015). Such an approach has been persuasive in influencing the Government Report on Transgender Equality (House of Commons Women's Equality Committee, 2016), whose conclusions feed into the forthcoming Gender Identity (Protected Characteristic) Bill 2016-2017.

The Government Report recommends a change in the protected characteristic under the Equality Act 2010 from 'gender reassignment' to 'gender identity'. Instead of requiring a diagnosis of gender dysphoria, a medical certificate of gender re-assignment, and to have lived as your chosen gender for a minimum of two years, an individual would simply be able to declare him or herself a man or woman and sign a statement of intention to live as such. This act, if implemented, will represent a fundamental shift in how we understand ourselves as humans: our sexual dimorphism, our reproductive biology and how, as women and men, our relations are organized for us within the public sphere. Hopefully, a movement of resistance will grow when the implications for women of this legal reform are finally realized.

With regard to children, the Government Report concludes that a new approach to caring for transgender children should be speedily implemented. Ironically, the shift from medicalized gender re-assignment to gender self-identification intensifies the call for medical intervention. Recommendations for a new approach include: reducing the amount of time required for the assessment that children must undergo before puberty blockers and cross-sex hormones can be prescribed; further provision of staff training in gender identity issues to be taught as part of PSHE classes in schools; a change in the application process for Gender Recognition Certificates to be based on 'self-declaration' in place of a diagnosis of gender dysphoria; the right of 'gender non-conforming' adolescents to have their 'true gender' recognized on the basis of self-determination; reducing the minimum age at which application can be made for gender recognition from 18 to 16; and an expansion of the definition of 'trans' to include the full spectrum gender variant, gender non-conforming, gender diverse or gender atypical identities (Transgender Trend, 2016a).

Transgender Trend (2016a) demonstrates the report manages to accomplish two seemingly contradictory things. Firstly, it normalizes the 'transgender child', since the meaningless array of genders she or he can choose potentially includes any child who doesn't conform to gender stereotypes. Vulnerable teenagers will be "especially susceptible to this 'pick your personality' self-classification choice". Secondly, the report 'others' children who don't fit gender stereotypes as requiring special medical treatment. With regard to lessening of the age at which youth can receive treatment, very little attention is paid to examining the underlying causes of children's 'will to transition', the pressures within teen culture to self-define as trans, or the physical effects on the body of medicalized transitioning (Transgender Trend, 2016a).

In conclusion, the figure of the real, incontrovertible and ahistorical 'transgender child' has taken less than 20 years to be complete. Broadly speaking over this period of time, young people have been offered two identities: the first is that of the unfortunate victim 'born in the wrong body' who requires medical diagnosis and treatment; the second is that of revolutionary self-identifying, 'non-binary' adolescent who bravely sensitizes the rest of us to the complexities and politics of gender. These seemingly opposed identities are still evolving and taking shape, but are increasingly synthesized into one. Where transgender lobbying and medicine originally brought 'the transgender child' into being, the law is now confirming and re-enforcing its 'reality'.

Conclusion

At the beginning of this chapter I argued 'the transgender child' emerged out of the knowledge-power-ethics relations of adult transgender doctrine and politics. Here I argue that the same strategies and tactics which shut down debate are also applied to feminists attempting to open public dialogue about the ethics of transgendering children.

The movement to transgender children reserves the right to create its own truths and moral values from within, and often responds with *ad hominem* slurs lodged at anyone who in good faith raises different possibilities of understanding. Gender critics are accused of bigotry, exercising 'cis' privilege, inciting hate speech, and/or they tarred with the epithet TERF. Whilst writing this chapter a fellow academic wrote by email that children are not harmed by the process of transgendering but, and I quote, by "the ignorance" of gender critical feminists like myself.

Parents and care-givers are "typically caught", she alleges, "between a range of unimaginably difficult situations and decisions, of which further judgement from others (typically Trans Exclusionary Radical Feminists, otherwise known as TERFs) is deeply harmful and not at all feminist". This is typical example of 'TERF' as "an anti-feminist shame-phrase, a speech-weapon of choice, a wedge noun used to splinter and insult gender critical feminists" (Craft, 2016).

As a male to female transsexual, Gender Apostate argues the transgender movement has been extremely successful in enabling transwomen to claim they are misunderstood and politically oppressed by 'cis' feminists (Gender Apostate, 2015). He (I use Gender Apostate's preferred pronoun) insists that it takes strength to transition and challenge gender norms, but, as someone who has found this strength, he insists transwomen challenge nothing if their actions maintain and reinforce the patriarchy. Nikki Craft, a political activist and writer, argues the transgender movement consistently attributes oppressive attitudes to radical feminists and systematically misrepresents feminist agendas and allegiances (Craft, 2016). The myth circulates that gender critical feminists wish to prevent individual adults from altering their bodies through biochemical or surgical means. Nothing could be further from the truth. Gender critical feminists are respectful of an individual's choice to transgender since basic human rights dictate that no-one should be discriminated against because of their choice of identity. Human beings self-create and have differing ideas about how to construct 'the self' (Murray, 2017). In a liberal society, it is imperative that self-construction is permitted "so long as no-one else is harmed in the process and so long as claims are not made on other people's resources to facilitate the individual's personal projects in self-design" (Murray, 2016: 2). Problems with transgenderism only emerge when political claims are made that have serious impact on the rights, freedoms and bodily integrity of other social groups.

In a relatively short period of time the cultural context for raising girls and boys has changed. In the 1970s and 1980s, the idea that gender is a social construct was the commonly accepted progressive model for raising children. Parents attempted to help their sons and daughters escape from gender binarism through assurance that there is *no* uniform way girls and boys necessarily feel, think and behave. This is the model of parenting that I deployed. One of my three sons, as a twelve-year-old, freely wore his sister's clothes at home for some months as he experimented with 'masculinity' and 'femininity' in his adolescent years. Why would his father and I suggest to him he might be a girl in his male body? Since the figure of the 'transgender child' had not yet been invented, our son grew up with his male body thankfully unharmed and, if you're interested, to be a heterosexual man.

Recently I shared a long train journey with a thoughtful friend who is the mother of a primary school-age boy and we discussed the construction of 'the transgender child'. Her son has beautiful long blond hair that she is reluctant to shorten and he loves wearing multi-coloured nail varnish on his toes. She consistently strives to carve out a 'gender-free zone' for him, but inevitably fails since children's lives are increasingly saturated by ideas about what it is to be a 'boy' or 'girl' – from the gendered marketing of children's toys and books, to the heroes and characters of cartoons, to the ideology of Gendered Intelligence in schools. Nevertheless, my friend found somewhat extreme the proposition that the 'transgender child' is an entirely socially constructed figure. "Surely", she worried, "although I would resist any attempt by his school or by Gendered Intelligence to suggest *my* son is a girl there *might* be some children who really *are* transgender?" Her anxiety illustrates how 'the transgender child' has become so embedded in the cultural imagination that its 'reality' is difficult to question, even by a parent critical of gender.

A future generation may look back with astonishment at the sheer moral and intellectual certitude that 'the transgender child' is real. Perhaps people will wonder why the obvious inconsistencies of the knowledge on whose grounds we accede children are 'born in the wrong body' were not questioned. Perhaps they will judge the present liberal moment which condones young people to make life-changing decisions that will affect their future lives in ways they can't possibly predict or understand as a derogation of societal responsibility. One day people may marvel that it became fashionable to evoke feminism, once a revolutionary political movement which rejected gender, to silence today's feminists when they continue to eschew it. Perhaps people will scrutinize whose interconnected interests were served by the numerous trans-led organizations which lobbied intensively for children to be accorded medico/legal rights to transgender. They may be astonished at the alacrity, even violence, with which, in a democratic society founded on free speech, discussion was foreclosed whenever public, collective debate of transgender doctrine was proposed. They may look back at the practice of transgendering children as an historical abuse that bizarrely happened in plain sight. I hope so.

References

American Psychological Association (2015) 'Guidelines for Psychological Practice with Transgender and Gender Nonconforming People', *American Psychologist*, 70(9), 832-864

Butler, J. (1990) *Gender Trouble*, Routledge: New York and London

—. (2004) *Undoing Gender*, Routledge: New York and London

Craft, N. (2016) http://www.theturfwarzone.com

De Beauvoir, S. (1949) (new edition 1997) *The Second Sex: Facts and Myths*, Vintage Classics: London

Department of Health (2008) *Medical Care for Gender Variant Children and Young People: Answering Families' Questions*, National Health Service, London. http://webarchive.nationalarchives.gov.uk/20101121114206/http://www.dh.gov.uk/prod_consum_dh/groups/dh_digitalassets/@dh/@en/documents/digitalasset/dh_082954.pdf

Eliot, L. (2010) *Pink Brain, Blue Brain: How Small Differences Grow Into Troublesome Gaps - And What We Can Do About It*, Mariner Books, New York: USA

Endocrine Society (2009) 'Endocrine Treatment of Transsexual Persons: An Endocrine Society Clinical Practice Guidelines', *The Journal of Clinical Endocrinology and Metabolism (JCEM)*: Chevy Chase

Fine, C. (2010) *Delusions of Gender: How our Minds, Society and Neuroscience Create Difference* W.W. Norton and Company: New York and London

—. (2017) *Testosterone Rex: Myths of Science, Sex, Science and Society*, W.W. Norton and Company: New York and London

Fine, C., Jordan-Young, R., Kaiser, A. and Rippon, G. (2013) 'Plasticity, plasticity, plasticity ... and the rigid problem of sex'. *Trends in Cognitive Sciences*, Vol. 17, No. 11, 11.2013, p. 550-551

Foucault, M. (1982) 'The Subject and Power' in Dreyfus, H. and Rabinow, P. (1982) *Michel Foucault: Beyond Structuralism and Hermeneutics*, Harvester Wheatsheaf: New York and London.

—. (1994) 'The Ethics of the Concern for the Self as a Practice of Freedom' in Rabinow, P. (ed.) *Michel Foucault: Ethics, The Essential Works of Foucault 1954-1984, Volume 1*, Penguin: London

Gender Apostate (2015) 'Cissexism and You' http://genderapostates.com/cissexism-and-you/

Gendered Intelligence (2017) http://genderedintelligence.co.uk

Gendered Intelligence Training (2017)
http://genderedintelligence.co.uk/professionals/therapists-and-counsellors
Gender Identity Research and Education Society (2017)
http://www.gires.org.uk
House of Commons Women's Equality Commission (2016) *Transgender Equality: First Report of Session 2015-2016*,
https://publications.parliament.uk/pa/cm201516/cmselect/cmwomeq/390/390.pdf
Izaakson, J. (2017) *The PWR BTTM Debacle Demonstrates Why Queer Politics Don't Protect Women Women*
http://www.feministcurrent.com/2017/05/23/pwr-bttm-debacle-demonstrates-queer-politics-dont-protect-women/
Jeffreys, S. (2014) *Gender Hurts: A Feminist Analysis of the Politics of Transgenderism*, Routledge: London and New York
Jensen, R. (2017) *The End of Patriarchy: Radical Feminism for Men*, Spinifex Press: Australia
Joel, D. (2016) 'Captured in Terminology: Sex, Sex Categories, and Sex Differences', Feminism & *Psychology*, 26, 335–345
Joel, D., Berman, Z., Wexler, N., Gaber, O., Stein, Y., Shefi, N. Pool, J., Urchs, S., Marguilies, D.S., Liem, F., Hanggi, J., Jancke, L. and Assaf, Y. (2015) 'Sex Beyond the Genitalia: The Human Brain Mosaic', *Proceedings of the National Academy of Science (PNAS)* November 2015, 112 (50).
Mermaids (2017) http://www.mermaidsuk.org.uk
Mort, F. (1987) *Dangerous Sexualities: Medico-Moralistic Politics in England Since 1830*, Routledge and Kegan Paul: London and New York
Murphy, M. (2017) *It's No Mystery Why the Queerest Generation Ever Hasn't Managed to Address Women's Oppression*
http://www.feministcurrent.com/2017/07/03/no-mystery-queerest-generation-ever-womens-oppression/
Murray, T. (2016) *Has 'Trans Rights' Become Homophobia's New Idiom?*
https://conatusnews.com/trans-rights-homophobia
—. (2017) *The Hijacking of Gender: A Feminist Take on Transgenderism*
http://www.cultureontheoffensive.com/hijacking-gender-feminist-take-transgenderism
Raymond, J. G. (1980) *The Transsexual Empire*, The Women's Press: London

Reilley-Cooper, R. (2016) *Gender is Not a Spectrum.*
https://sociologie.uqam.ca/upload/files/activites/2016-11-04%20rebecca_reilly-cooper_coll_societe.pdf

Royal College of General Practitioners (RCGP) (2017) *Gender Variance E-Learning Module.*
http://elearning.rcgp.org.uk/gendervariance

Stewart, J. (2015) *We Are Living on the Cusp of a Gender Revolution*
https://www.youtube.com/watch?

—. (2017) *Trans Youth Are Real.*
https://genderedintelligence.wordpress.com

Tavistock Announcement (2017) *GIDS referrals increase slows in 2016/17*
https://tavistockandportman.nhs.uk/about-us/news/stories/gids-referrals-increase-slows-201617

Transgender Trend (2015) *Welcome to Transgender Trend*
https://www.TransgenderTrend.com/surprising-referrals-children-tavistock-clinic-continue-soar

—. (2016) *Parents Question New Government Report*
https://www.TransgenderTrend.com/surprising-referrals-children-tavistock-clinic-continue-soar

—. (2016a) *UK Government Report on Transgender Equality*
https://www.TransgenderTrend.com/surprising-referrals-children-tavistock-clinic-continue-soar

—. (2017) *Stonewall School Report: What Does The 45% Attempted Suicide Rate Really Mean?* https://www.TransgenderTrend.com/stonewall-school-report-what-does-suicide-rate-mean

—. (2017a) *Is It Surprising That Referrals of Children to the Tavistock Clinic Continue to Soar?* https://www.TransgenderTrend.com/surprising-referrals-children-tavistock-clinic-continue-soar

Weeks, J. (1985) *Sexuality and Its Discontents: Meanings, Myths and Modern Sexualities*, Routledge and Kegan Paul: London and Boston

CHAPTER FOUR

'I'M NOT A HIDEOUSLY BIGOTED PARENT WHO DOESN'T 'GET' IT'

GENDERCRITICALDAD

Why I'm writing

I'm not an expert, not a psychologist or a social worker or a child development specialist. I'm not a writer or a journalist. I'm an inexperienced writer. I failed my English at school and had to retake my exams. I'll get into my reasons for writing later.

  I'm contributing to this book because I started a blog *http://GenderCriticalDad.blogspot.co.uk* which gained far more attention that I ever imagined possible. In this chapter I draw on some of what I've written for my blog. I feel really that I am a bit of a fraud contributing my blog to the internet and now this chapter to the book. I have no humanities education, beyond reading loads of books when I was younger. Writing is painful for me. I'll take a break from writing to pull my nose hairs out. I have no experience of 'doing' politics and feel I can barely string a coherent argument together. What is really surprising is that these days readers value my arguments. People quote me as a source or rely on material I've posted. I can't deny that it's immensely flattering to find I have readers. People have used things I've said as mottos for their blogs, or quoted me on Twitter suggesting I might be building some real depth of knowledge and informed opinion.

  I write my blog in part, because it's better than having a chest full of feelings that I can't make sense of as a parent with a daughter who says she wants to be a man. If I can write my confusions down it becomes easier to understand myself. I write the blog in part, to let other people know they are not alone if they question trans dogma. My personal story seems to have connected with some people and sometimes helped them, which is just so good. I write the blog in part to contribute to the cause of transcritical thinking; 'defeating the Transgender doctrine and the dogma of Gender Identity' I mean.

Who I am and how life used to be

I'm a middle of the road dad. Lefty liberal newspaper reader, organic eggs and chicken, equal shares sort of dad. Probably I'm a bit insensitive, a bit impatient and definitely a bit lazy. I earn my living making machines do stuff for people, or fixing them when they don't work. To do that you keep an eye out for the difference between how people think things are and how they really are. You might think a fault is caused by one component failing, but you must check it to be sure you've fixed it. People might say they want the machine to do one thing, but until you start to build a prototype and see if it works you have no certainty that they actually know it can do what they want it to do. In my work, I find people frequently see the world as they wish it was and see me as being a difficult techie when I try to explain that the world might be otherwise and the machine they have in mind might not be the machine I can build. So I am used to thinking critically and trying to explain alternative thinking.

Up until around a year ago, things were alright at home. My daughter was always a quiet, smart kid. When she puts her mind to something, she's very determined. If she encounters unfairness, she fights it head on. She had no clue about how to manipulate people.

A couple of years ago she came out to us as a lesbian, after dropping countless clues. We were totally unsurprised, had been wondering when she would tell us. She started dressing quite 'butch' which was no problem. Who wants to go out in shoes that hurt and uncomfortable clothes that restrict you? She cut her hair short which I thought was a good idea as she never could be bothered to brush it and she has a lovely long neck and bone structure that short hair shows off well. Years ago I'd worked with several lesbians. They had been great people to work with. We were all young, we all had our dramas, but overall they tended to be a bit less undignified than straight people. I could imagine my daughter fitting in well with the lesbian crowd. Smart, pretty with a bit of attitude, she would have been very popular.

Ignoring the Warnings

My daughter started becoming fascinated with drag queens.

She started getting at me and my partner for not being like 'normal' mums and dads. We are very boring, unexciting people she thinks, but it really wound her up that in her view we don't particularly fit in with sexist stereotypes for parents. I'm a dad who hates football and big cars and likes cooking; her mum never wears make up, has short hair, rarely wears a dress and hates cooking. It isn't that we are some sort of 'super right on' couple. I'm way too lazy about housework and, to be honest, don't do my share. How we are is just how we are.

My daughter's butch dress code became more extreme and more compulsive. She decided it was no longer OK to wear man-ish clothes or shoes; they had to be specifically men's clothes. Her bras were all replaced with sport bras and then she started wearing a binder. We tried not to react. I remember I dressed like a fright at her age and could imagine why going out with a bust might be awkward for a teenage girl. She dropped hints about transgender, nothing specific, just a bit of Social Justice Warrior talk that lots of teenagers come out with. In her small group of school friends people seemed to be changing sexual orientation all the time. Then 'gender identity' became the latest trendy thing and she talked about it more. Her mum and I decided to just ignore it, wait for the next trend to come by and pass over. She started going to a Gender Support Group which I imagined to be a bit like a lesbian feminist consciousness raising group where she could sit round discussing how much men screw over women and what a dinosaur her dad is.

One evening we went to a parents' evening at her school. A teacher told us how much she liked our child and how well they got on and how she, the teacher, had made our daughter a new name badge with a boy's name and now used our daughter's preferred pronouns. The situation was getting surreal but we let it ride thinking 'our girl has important exams coming up' 'she's under so much pressure nowadays', 'she's had ups and downs at school and doesn't need any more drama, just let it ride'.

Hitting Peak Trans

Then one night we went out for a family meal. Lovely place, great food. Our daughter started talking about how much better life will be when she reaches eighteen and can start taking Testosterone and have top surgery. Now remember, I'm the sort of bloke who people laugh at for being a liberal type, opting for free range organic chicken, always voting Labour. I've always supported LGB rights, just because I think it right and just that lesbian, gay and bisexual people have the same rights as everyone else, it makes sense. I didn't think anything of it when the Trans got added creating LGBT - thinking 'trans is just more gay' right?

But this? This was about surgery, removing healthy tissue to fix something called 'gender dysphoria'. My daughter was now talking about spending her lifetime on an artificial hormone regime. I was supposed to go along with this? Ignore the memory of being with her since birth as a baby girl through being a little girl then growing into a young woman. What she was saying now suddenly got very scary. Talk of a lifetime on untested hormones seemed to be madness and I felt I was being asked to accept something that was very wrong. What had made my wonderful daughter decide on a course of self-mutilation and lifelong drug dependency?

I felt I was expected to support her on this difficult journey to a 'bright new gender fluid future'. I knew this was the new modern trans-accepting prescription that the BBC, the leading liberal newspaper The Guardian, our schools and the NHS were promoting as the cure for the latest children's malady: gender dysphoria. I just couldn't go along with this direction. It seemed my daughter had given up on being herself and in doing so was betraying generations of women who had fought for women's and lesbian rights. Her ideas about her identity and her future were full of contradictions, full of danger for her and would leave her living a lie. But everywhere we turned the social expectation seemed to be we should support or even celebrate our daughter's trans identification with all its requirements for off-label drugs and a double mastectomy; this was simply the next step to go along with in giving full acceptance of the rights of LGBTQ people; acceptance of our daughter's identification as transgender was held out as an essential liberating act and proper affirmation of who our daughter really was. I wondered if I was losing my balance and ability to adapt, my sanity was unravelling or was I just a hideously bigoted old-fashioned dad in a minority of one?

Doubting Myself

Was I thinking about my daughter being transgender like a rigid bigot? Was I transphobic? The only people who seemed to share my worries about transgender identity were women writers like Germaine Greer, being labelled a dinosaur by feminists (Welsh, 2015) and transphobic and a TERF (Lewis, 2015) by the liberal and conservative press, who everyone it seemed now agreed had lost the plot. Or worse, am I thinking like a religious bigot, who really hates people who aren't heterosexual because they think it says to do so in the bible?

I found myself at odds with every cultural fixture in my world. Everyone around me seemed to accept the idea that my daughter could become a man as the new truth. I needed to know more, to understand more. Before all this kicked off with my own daughter, my image of transgender people conjured up either wildly flamboyant drag queens or awkward people who don't really fit in as occasionally portrayed in a television soap opera.

I'd always understood drag queens to be making jokes out of femininity, turning a joke on uptight straight men "you fancy me, but I'm a man", a sexual fetish, both in doing it and in chasing "chicks with dicks". Yes drag queens can be funny I suppose, they can challenge straight male sexuality and well, whatever floats your boat. I know some women object to drag queens because the line between parodying femininity and being misogynist is a fine line and often overstepped but that was never really something that affected me. I really hadn't previously thought much about transgender. If asked about a transgender woman I would have thought of her as a woman who just happened to have a past as a man. I hadn't thought much about what her genital arrangements were but this wouldn't have mattered to me - if the person seemed happy what was there to object to?

Diving into Trans

I now had to think and learn fast because my daughter was telling me she was transgender and intended to be a man. I googled frenetically and found a disquieting world. A newspeak of Assigned Male At Birth (Gender Wiki, undated), of trans woman, but never transwoman (Taking Up Too Much Space, 2008). Of how gender is nothing to do with sexuality, of pronouns (Lesbian, Gay, Bisexual, Transgender Resource Centre, undated) and suicide (Malone, 2015) and transphobia and cis privilege (Dylan-Finch, 2016) and thousands of trans women murdered (National LGBTQ Taskforce, 2016) because of the transphobia spread by dreadful Trans Exclusionary Radical Feminists (Adams, 2017). I started to wonder about TERFs (White, 2015). Researching further I found out that the whole transgender phenomenon was not quite as I had assumed. I discovered most male to trans people (MtT) have not, and many do not intend to have surgery, had started out as straight men and later identified as lesbian or bisexual trans women (Quora, undated). This somehow didn't fit in with the 'gayer than gay' idea. I found out that most female to trans (FtT) people started out as Lesbian women who had identified as 'butch' before transitioning but that a side effect of taking testosterone was to make them attracted to men (Godfrey, 2015).

When I looked at transgender websites I found a similar asymmetry. There were young men looking like would-be drag queens with either a pout from a porn trope or a stroppy sneer reminiscent of a punk band looking like they reject all things suburban (Instagram, 2017). Old blokes looking like old blokes in a frock (Strudwick, 2016). I saw the same insistence on all transactivist websites that everyone accept men as women full stop. I read articles instructing that saying male to trans people are 'men' is 'literally' an act of violence (Dennis, 2017).

I found feminist websites insisting 'trans women are women' whatever they look like and that non-trans women must accept transwomen as real women (Dennis, 2017a). I discovered that women who aren't transwomen have something called 'cis-privilege' because they never question their gender, nor have it questioned and that this makes them less oppressed than trans women (Williams, 2014). Apparently, according to Wikipedia , cis-women don't suffer from gender dysphoria, "the dysphoria (distress) a person experiences as a result of the sex and gender they were assigned at birth" - a claim which in no way fits the struggle all my female friends have dealt with all their lives.

I discovered that thousands of years of sexist oppression was immaterial to the rights of cis-women and their fear of rape will have to be ignored to allow transwomen with penises to be in the space of cis women. I read that any mention of female biology, menstruation or contraception was transphobic and would 'trigger' men identifying as women (MtT's) perhaps leading to suicide because trans women feel excluded from the biology of non-trans womanhood. And mention of female biology, menstruation or contraception was also transphobic I came to understand because it would 'trigger' women identifying as men (FtTs) by drawing unwanted attention to their female biology.

I learned how the life of transgender people can be made unbearable by someone using the wrong pronouns or 'dead-naming' - referring to a transgender person's birth name instead of their chosen name. According to the sites I was reading the rights of transgender women must trump the rights of cis-women to have their own spaces for safety, comfort, dating or just to talk and think together (Ginelle, 2015). I learned how the long-running award-winning feminist play *The Vagina Monologues* is now viewed as exclusionary and must be banned because of the hurt it causes to women without vaginas and men with vaginas (Mulhere, 2015). How a health training exercise making cupcakes iced to look like vulvas, intended as a genuine attempt to educate people about the many shapes of healthy women's body parts, was hateful and exclusionary and triggering and would no doubt kill trans people (Glick, 2015).

I went along to a Parents of Trans Young People meeting, put on by a national gender identity organisation. There I met a group of eight or so nervous looking young people aged between twelve and eighteen years all sitting hunched up and uneasy with eyes downcast. Sweets and crisps were provided for the young ones. Parents were all looking terrified. The meeting was facilitated by two transwomen. One looked, frankly, like the someone from the English comedy television series *League of Gentlemen* featuring bizarre townsfolk all played by (biological) men, not scary, just anxious. The other facilitator was less ridiculous. He was tall, 6ft 1" or more, strapping lad, early twenties, carrying a few pounds on his hips and growing 'moobs' to resemble a woman's breasts. The immediate dislike between us was mutual. This character, a biological male, had apparently been a woman all his life but recently started transition. Prior to identifying as transgender he had fathered a child and had an ex-wife. He was now a butch lesbian transwoman. A 6'1" fifteen stone lesbian with hands like a blacksmith and size twelve feet. This person spent their time counselling confused young people about sex and gender. The meeting kicked off with a little talk about respect and pronouns and not being hurtful and how we should all show respect by using the right pronouns and to help us with this we would do a 'pronoun circle' exercise each saying what name we wanted to be called and what pronouns we wanted used to refer to us. Everyone present played the pronoun game. No one wanted to be rude, or ignorant or disrespectful.

Online, I carried on with my research. I learned about the 'cotton ceiling' a term used by trans porn star and activist Drew DeVeaux to refer to lesbians refusing to have sex with people with penises, arguably a bigoted and transphobic refusal. I learned how penises are not male (Serano, 2004) and vaginas are not female (The Nurse Path, 2017).

Looking for a Sane View

I read hundreds of posts on the Gender Critical subs on Reddit and all the links off the sidebars and found lots of apparently sane people, some of whom had been through the same sort of thing as me with their children. Some were professionals allied to education, health care, psychology and counselling, all trying to find a way to get a transcritical word out without losing their jobs. I found out just how sinister and wide ranging the transgender agenda was, that other people had realised it was woman hating and the view that transgender activism promotes the opposite of gay and lesbian liberation is widespread. Transgender activism could eradicate gays and lesbians in a generation (Vabvox, 2015). Eviscerate feminism and reframe the reality of women's oppression to a bad consumer choice.

I found a sane and respectable, professional philosopher, Rebecca Reilly-Cooper and her blog 'More Radical with Age' written with an illuminating clarity that normal non-academic people can follow. She pulled the core of the transgender dogma to pieces like a DIY car manual, leaving it spread out with all the contradictions in plain sight (Reilly-Cooper, 2016). I found Maria Catt (Catt, undated) and 4th Wave (4thWaveNow, undated), Purple Sage (Purple Sage, undated) and YouthTransCriticalProfessionals (YouthTransCriticalProfessionals, undated) and many more transcritical voices all telling different transcritical stories, all showing a different side to transgender orthodoxy, all describing a world richer and way more complex than the simplistic dogma that gender dysphoria is when the gender of your brain does not match the sex of your body and the cure is to transition.

Keeping secrets, being hated, hoping and waiting

I believe 'good parents' love their children. They want the best for them. They want them to grow into independent, happy adults. 'Good parents' accept that their children have to choose their own way, make their own decisions and learn from their own mistakes. As the children grow nearer to adulthood, they may offer guidance but 'good parents' never give orders. Sometimes even the children of 'good parents' make bad choices and those choices threaten their permanent wellbeing. If these choices involve serious drug abuse, crime, abusive relationships or mental illness, there are support groups, interventions, *Al-Anon, Nar-Anon, S-Anon* and mental health systems and therapies.

People I know tend to accept that when children hit adolescence they may well rebel, hate their parents and rage at them. Society and friends will support families, understanding that the parents are seeing the bigger picture and have their young one's best interests at heart. Friends and family and school and the family friendly doctor will usually empathise with hard choices having to be made and reassure parents that they are doing the right thing trying to put in place boundaries for their child's well-being. When your child falls under the spell of transgender none of this happens.

Your children will say they hate you. They will tell you that only surgery and drugs will make their life bearable. They will say you are an evil hateful person for not helping them down the path laid out for them towards a bright new progressive world of transgender. You will feel utterly alone. In the case of your child saying they are transgender, the media, politicians, rock stars, your child's school and those family friendly health services will all tell you that you must support your child by agreeing to whatever the child feels they need to do to become a person of the opposite gender. To do anything else, to talk to your child about your worries for them, to gently ask questions, to try to explain biology to your own child, is to show what a bigoted, prejudiced and transphobic person you are. In the UK, you, the caring, questioning, reflective careful parent, are told you will be to blame if your child self-harms or commits suicide (Peoples Trust Toronto, 2014).

You must keep your worries secret for the sake of your child's privacy and to avoid confrontations that will push you child away. You must protect your friends and extended family from the grief of knowing your child's trans identity is extremely dangerous and shield others from having to pick sides. You must face the well-meaning parents of your child's friends. They will mostly be smug and use your child's new name and pronouns. They will inwardly congratulate themselves on how progressive they are ignoring their own eyes and memory. You will see the flash of liberal revulsion on their faces when you don't join in and instead use the name that you have used for *your child,* for the whole of *your child's* life.

Finding a Way to Cope

I had to keep some relationship going with my daughter without giving in to the insane demands of her transitioning and somehow avoid confrontation. I had to weather her rages and sulks bottling down my own anger and hurt. I did everything I could think of to draw my daughter back to reality and to set up situations where we could do something together that makes me feel like a normal parent and where she and I can be happy together. That's all I can do: Keep as much of a relationship going as I can and wait and hope for reality to reassert itself. You can't argue with a closed mind shored up by a cult ideology. Trying to reason will only reinforce delusional beliefs, push my daughter further into the transgender cult. You can't play therapist. Living with a transitioning child is not like portrayed in films of infinite family wisdom and courage and there will be no dramatic reconciliation with tears and hugs and easy recovery. I'm not a therapist. I mess about with machines for a living, but I will now go on to describe how my partner and I try to deal with day to day life. Our approach is not original; it's an extrapolation of some standard ways of dealing with problematic behaviour in people that we have clung on to as a set of strategies for coping:

Ignore:
Don't mention trans and don't argue about trans. Don't rise to any provocation. Don't be dramatic about this and don't make a point of ignoring it. Don't say you're ignoring it just quietly get on with doing something else. Teenagers can be difficult anyway so try not to see everything in terms of trans; sometimes trans teenagers are just being teenagers.

Redirect:
Do something else with your trans child that is good for both of you and nothing to do with trans. Again, don't make a point about it and don't state why you're doing it. Just think of something you can do together which has nothing to do with trans, but that will be something they can join in with. It can be something that seems really small, choosing what to have for tea, choosing something on Netflix to watch together. It doesn't have to be a worthy or anti-trans activity.

Reward:
Be positive for anything but trans. Don't make a big point of it, don't mention trans, just be nice about whatever your child does that isn't trans related.

Implementing the above plan is not always easy. It means you must ignore a lot of hateful talk and behaviour. You must let it wash over you and yes it will sometimes get to you. Find a friend you can talk to, go for a run, do some DIY, phone a help-line or write an anonymous blog: you are the adult, you have to deal with your transitioning child.

Caring for Myself

These days I know I'm not alone and that my instinctive critical reaction to trans does not make me a bigot. Other, sane, wise and humane people - such as fellow contributors to this book - have come to the same conclusions as me and are equally worried about transgender activism directed at children and young people. In our family, my child's mother and I have a strategy to do our absolute best for our daughter and not collude with the false promises of those who tell her she can turn into a man. In general our approach seems to be buying time. We have good days, we have times together when we share laughs with our daughter, days when she can live in her body and be OK with it, particularly such days if we can get her away from transactivists and the internet.

But life with a transitioning teenager is unbelievably difficult. My daughter, one of the people most precious to me, is still walking towards the cliff edge of attaining adulthood with a head full of nonsense and lies telling her that she is a man born in the body of a woman and that her perception of her gender is what makes her a man or a woman. Transgender activism tells her that if she changes her name and takes some medicine and has significant surgery she can become a man as real as any other man. Transgender activism tells my daughter the rest of the world must agree with her perception and does her an injustice if they do not. Anyone who questions the dogma or the wisdom of her decisions exposes themselves as an evil bigot and she must be mindful of this. My daughter is being damaged by transgender dogma and simultaneously represents that dogma in my life. I hate what it's doing to her, but I love her. I cannot attack transgender dogma without harming her. I must deftly ignore reproach when she throws it in my face. I must smoothly change the situation to focus on something positive and then concentrate on that positivity and reflect it back to her. This is the only strategy I have for resisting transgender ideas. Staying calm and quietly moving over contentious things my child is saying doesn't come naturally to me. I'm a grumpy old bloke. Sometimes I mess up. I find myself and my daughter screaming and shouting at each other. The 'Ignore, Redirect and Reward' mantra flies out of the window and clash of the dogmas takes over. This is not helpful.

I needed a way to fight transactivism away from my daughter. However ineffective, however pathetic, I had to do something with the energy and rage spiralling round my head. I invented GenderCriticalDad and created a blog for him. He can say what I cannot. GenderCriticalDad can reach out and connect with other parents, talk with lesbians and radical feminists and discuss ideas with anyone who questions the doctrine of gender identity. GenderCriticalDad has to be separate from the real me, untraceable. Some details are blurred in my writing, some changed, so that even if my daughter finds her way to the GenderCriticalDad blog she won't recognise the two of us.

A kind soul from Reddit helped me with my first post, 'way too many commas', 'get that spelling sorted', 'post it and put a note on reddit / Gender Critical to tell people about it'. Nowadays I can get into a sort of method for coping through writing. Some experience or observation sparks off an idea and winds me up. I write some notes, unstructured, ungrammatical, leave what I've written for a couple of days, rearrange the notes in to some sort of order. Come back, drink plenty of coffee, smoke too much, write the story out as I would speak it, try to keep the piece as concise as possible, read it out aloud as I go, does it scan like me talking? Leave it. Come back the next day and tidy it up, cut anything that's rubbish. Writing a blog to exorcise the pain of living with a transitioning child, to expose confusion, to promote discussion. To unravel strategies that might protect daughters like mine and family's like yours from the grip of the cult of transgender.

Some people like the blog. Many parents say they recognise experiences and agonies in their own lives. Writing the GenderCriticalDad blog feels of some help to people and evidently makes a connection with other traumatised and panicking parents. Some of what I write is rephrasing ideas from other people, trying to spread ideas from radical feminism to people like myself, ordinary blokes who might not come across certain writers. Some of my writing consists just of me blurting out distress that I need to get out. People like the telling the truth of the agony more; sharing experience touches people, perhaps offering them solace or sometimes a bit of hope. Most of the comments I receive on the blog are encouraging people offering support or just saying 'me too'. I pick up a couple of trolls. One is a trans woman who tries to draw me into debates. Another transwoman repeatedly tells me I'll be sorry for transcritical thinking when my son kills himself.

Connecting and Solidarity

So far the story in this chapter has been all about me trying to survive on my own with connection only to strangers struggling with transgender children I found via the internet.

One day another parent contacted me. There's this thing about sceptical parents of trans identifying kids. We are all paranoid as hell. There are aggressors out there, pouty lads, proudly pictured with half an inch of Max Factor Photoshop, a bit of lippy and a knife or a baseball bat underneath death threat slogans in garish type aimed at parents who question the truth of transgenderism. The last thing your trans child needs is to have a parent who is outed as a TERF. If your child found out you were public about your concerns they would tell their mates just how oppressed they are by their TERF parents. And they would probably tell their teachers too who would collude in determining you are your own child's oppressor. Your child, faced with a transcritical parent, would be forced to choose between diving headlong into transition or being outcast from the cult they have become dependent on. Parents who work in related professions who don't believe the trans dogma have to be immensely careful, or they will lose their jobs and then be no longer able to help the children or students they teach, or support patients and clients they have known for years.

So, a parent who had been reading my blog made contact to ask if I want to be involved in talking to the press about our experience as transcritical parents. There might be an opportunity to get a gender critical view across and as GenderCriticalDad I could offer a way of putting gender critical views out without these always coming from a stereotyped feminist. I arrange to meet my fellow parent in secret at a motorway service station at night. I walk through the concessions between WH Smiths the newspaper outlet and Costa Coffee. I phone my contact and she's the ordinary woman standing three yards away from me. For transcritical parents to meet up we have to act like we're in a spy story written by comics and authors of best-selling thrillers. Two ordinary parents in England terrified of being outed as transcritical but knowing they must work together to protect their children and everybody else's from certain harm.

We talk for hours, coffee after coffee, finding huge relief at last each being able to speak to someone face to face going through the same transgender hell. I learn there is a group of people in regular internet contact with each other, some are parents of trans teenagers like myself, some are professionals working with children and young people, some happen to be both. I learn the group is meeting up for the first time in a Midlands town in a few weeks' time and then going on to a Feminist Event focussing on transgender in London. Do I want in? Hell Yes! It was so good to find people coming together to try and fight transgender dogma. So now I had a community of others, as well as my blog space where I can go when things get unbearable and just let my feelings out, not worrying about the world seeing me falling to pieces.

The press interview falls through when we refuse to expose our children's schools to the journalist who it turned out was seeking a salacious splash without a genuine care for anonymity of our daughters. A while later a small group of us working together manage to get Mariella Frostrup to say the words 'Gender Critical' on BBC Radio 4 (Frostrup, 2017) which was a tremendous breakthrough in a world of gender critical silence. But then my input to the same programme was twisted by a biased panel of discussants combined with BBC editorial cowardice. I quickly learn how scared the media are of encountering the wrath of the trans lobby. Our BBC contact tells us if media organisations don't tow the transgender line they receive death threats and hundreds of complaints accusing them of hate crime towards LGBT people (Saxby, undated).

Beginnings of resistance

The group of transcritical parents and professionals met in the Midlands town in an academics meeting room on a leafy campus. Some flew in especially from the US. I came face to face with people whose thoughtful transcritical blogs I read and reread, whose writing reached me when I was doubting my sanity and distrusting my own sense of decency. I was meeting people I felt were my s/heroes. I was overwhelmed by the collective wisdom in the room, the amazing writers and think I talked rather a lot. My transcritical allies were reflective people who took me and my GenderCriticalDad contribution seriously. We talked for several days finding much common ground, sharing our stories, thinking about collective action to break the transgender dogma our children are caught up by. We settled on writing this book. But more importantly we knew we all existed, were not mad, just ordinary people who didn't believe the transgender dogma and who would be prepared to stand together and say so.

The next day we travelled to London. Transcritical speakers assembled as *Feminists Thinking Differently* were among the finest thinkers of the radical feminist world (Murphy, 2016). Not tyrannical, man hating, fierce, haranguing activists but warm and funny commentators, rigorously laying into trans ideology and dogma, standing up for free speech, serious about women's rights and about protecting at all costs the rights of children to just be ordinary little original kids and sometimes confused children and young people like all children and young people are; the right to be whoever they wanted to be without being manipulated, drugged and mutilated. The *Feminists Thinking Differently* crowd was astonishing to me. I'm really a boring straight dad, middle aged, get up go to work, come home, make tea, wash up go to bed, get up again sort of bloke. I'd never seen such a diverse crowd of women, all content in their skin, not caring what men think of them and willing to include me. The strength and solidarity in this meeting was incredible and I began to believe transcritical activism could prevail.

I have to be undercover, strictly GenderCriticalDad, no one must know the real me is there, particularly my daughter must never know. Going to radical feminist events and collaborating with other people to bring down the trans orthodoxy would really betray the whole 'ignore redirect and reward' thing and I could lose my daughter. So wherever I go I avoid cameras, I hassle the photographer, trying to explain why I can't be photographed, not sure if they believe me. This is all a bit weird because while I was very paranoid about being identified I also knew that my daughter would love this bunch, she would feel at home even as a gender confused person and they would love and welcome her.

Meeting with Trans People

Soon after this, I was invited to another meeting called *Changing the Conversation* organised to bring feminists and trans people together to start a dialog. Someone suggested I might benefit from meeting some of the people going. I knew that Julie Bindel, the most notorious and frequently 'no-platformed' feminist in Britain was going, and some trans people I'd seen on the internet who had interesting views. I'd seen Bindel speak at the London event and was looking forward to meeting her but was really worried about meeting trans people. One of the trans people, Miranda Yardley, had been active on Twitter and had taken a lot of flak from trans activists. I thought we probably would agree on a lot but really I didn't know how I would react when meeting face to face. Meeting a transgender person was still outside of my experience. Now I have a chapter here in the same book as Miranda which shows that a wide range of transcritical perspectives have finally come together (this volume).

It turned out that Miranda Yardley and Julie Bindel had worked together before and are old mates. The notorious TERF and the "Transgender-non-conformant pomophobic transsexual" swapped obscene jokes and had obvious mutual shared affection. Miranda told us a bit of his story. He explained he did not fit the dominant trans narrative of being "a woman in a man's body". He simply wanted to live as he did without telling anyone what pronouns they should use. I think of Miranda as 'he' but I think that is as much to do with Miranda's terrible taste for prog rock music as anything else. Miranda doesn't give a damn about pronouns. We talked about how he has no wish to change his birth certificate, because that would be denying his past, which is part of him. He can also rock a goth dress with the best of them. He had an inspiring love for women and a wish to listen and learn from women. He vehemently objects to the silencing of people like Julie Bindel, he totally understands why women need the own spaces.

I spoke to Helen, another transwoman. She passes totally, not as a glammed up parody of femininity but as a straightforward middle aged woman with a sad note to her eyes when she thinks you're not looking.

Her story is complicated, not without regret, but involved times when transition was the only visible way forward. I also spoke with a butch woman dressed impeccably, shirt pressed perfectly, very dapper, very handsome, quiet but with immense presence, and a warmth and way of listening that I can't help but associate almost exclusively with women. She could have passed as a man but chose not to. She too just wanted to be what she was, live and dress how she liked. She and her conventionally gorgeous girlfriend made a wonderful couple. We talked about transmen and how a lot of her friends had transitioned, her sadness about that but her acceptance of their decisions. How she could see why they thought transitioning to be the best way for them at the time.

This is what I really learned from that day: some trans people, a lot of trans people, make their decision to transition *because that's the best option available to them at the time.* Everyone's story is different, every personal story is complicated. No experience I have encountered so far is really covered by the trans narrative. The trans people I have met don't want to dictate to anyone what they should think or say. They don't want to invade other people's spaces. They just want to live their lives as they are in whichever ways make them comfortable.

Choice, Possibilities and Who You Are

At the time of writing, my daughter is at a stage of life where she has all her choices laid out in front of her. It should be a great time full of exciting possibilities. I think she's decided the world of make-up and centring herself around men and boys is not for her. She may be attracted to women, she may not, but I don't think she identifies with the vision of sexuality offered by either the world of women's magazines or the world of porn. That makes sense to me, that's a healthy distance.

All the straight boys my daughter knows are porn sick. They have had smart phones since 2010. Ever present through their puberty, always two minutes and a few clicks away from the jackhammer, grim faced business of adult sexuality. That has comprised their sex education. That is what they think is real sex. Real men fuck hard, real men master the game of dominance and degradation, they smash it and wreck it. They may be crude and obvious, part of rape culture, or they may be sophisticated and keep a veneer of support for sex positive, inclusive non-shaming feminism. Whatever: men are in charge. It's serious and it's all about fucking hard. Women's pleasure is indistinguishable from women's pain and all comes from powerful, pounding penetration (Brunskell-Evans, 2016; Jensen, 2016, Jensen 2017).

If there are lesbians in this world of porn kids see, they are merely 'fluffers', waiting for the main event. Liberal feminism tells lesbians that they are transphobic and bigoted (Babcock, 2015). Identifying as a lesbian is nowadays just not cool, its old (Keating, 2017). When my daughter looks at the world what alternatives can she see? The one that at the moment makes most sense to her is the world of trans.

If she is a transman, or some flavour of 'trans lite', 'non-binary' whatever, she can step outside porn sick culture that diminishes girls like her. She can be queer, she can have some hope of a sexuality that is not totally centred on hard penetrative sex. I'm convinced she has alighted upon a false hope, leading to a cycle of dysphoria, and a different set of roles, but I can see how she might have come to this view.

There are women who can offer a different vision of the future for young women like my daughter. Lesbians, some who have been lesbians all their lives, some who have loved men and now love women, some loud and political lesbians, some just getting on with a quiet life. Feminists offer her hope, real feminists - 'the difficult kind' not apologists trying to make feminism acceptable to men and inclusive to whatever men want to do. Ordinary women who just don't have time or inclination for the whole femininity performance can be an inspiration to girls like mine. Women who have more important things in their life than worrying about gender tyranny. Women raising kids, women pursuing careers. Women being women according to women.

Women are diverse; they are the people who keep things running. Some are extraordinary some are ordinary. They are becoming invisible. They are not typically reality TV stars or featured in the glammed up word of celebrity. If transcritical women are visible they are dismissed as nasty, assumed to be 'white feminists', their voices are silenced because they are accused of having have cis-privilege by the transgender community. Transcritical women give me hope. Hope that by being there and getting seen they can offer a different future to my daughter.

Being Me and GenderCriticalDad

These days my life seems split into parts; walls of secrets delimiting each part and twisting me into contorted pieces. There is a lot of transcritical work I want to do that has to be put aside to talk rubbish about the telly with my daughter. Because actually that is the best thing I can do for her as her Dad and the most important thing I do right now. In life with my family, I pretend to be normal, not mentioning trans, trying to keep thing ordinary, showing love for my daughter and sustaining a normal life in actions and habits. In my family life I am a so-so dad, getting meals cooked, washing up, shopping, taking people places and fetching them back, taking the bins out.

Occasionally family life blows up, arguments and resentments explode. Resolutions are made and soon forgotten. Ideas of what I should do to save my daughter from the trans future of lifelong medication and irreversible surgery race round my head followed by a slamming wave of fear of how her life could all go terribly wrong. I should confront her, argue the transcritical case. I should make her read accounts of detranistioners, get her to watch trans regret videos, force her to confront the darks side of transactivism. I should sit down and ask her to just tell me how things got this way, re-establish real connection and use long forgotten skills to just listen, not correct, not argue just listen, listen, listen.

Insisting on a transcritical dialogue is much more terrifying than just carrying on day to day. The downside risk of a transcritical conversation is enormous. Life is bearable at the moment. I mustn't break the truce else I might lose my daughter. Sometimes I think things are maybe getting better, just hang on in, build her up, show love, living love. Please god let her peak trans be as painless as possible. Let's face it, if I was a better dad I wouldn't be here writing this. I have my own sexism, my own selfishness, my own anger. It seems to me I have failed to adequately listen to my daughter. I have somehow failed to hear the pain of trying to fit herself in the role of woman was causing her. I have failed to realize that her gender related pain was real, not imagined. Perhaps I have failed to show her, in love and actions not lectures, that she is great as she is. As GenderCriticalDad my aim is to make amends. She is completely wonderful as she is.

The hours with just me and my partner, just being normal, a time to rest from trans and not be on online, a chance to tell each other we are still good people, to share my undercover work, steal ideas from her or check that something I'm about to say isn't really feeble, are so precious and essential to carrying on.

The on-line version of GenderCriticalDad offers the edited best parts of my ongoing attempts to survive as the distraught dad of a daughter caught up in the cult of transgender, telling my story for others so that perhaps we each feel less alone or can sometimes stir things up or sometimes just play for sympathy. If you read GenderCriticalDad then you see someone way nicer than the guy sat here typing.

Being GenderCriticalDad has enabled me to learn so much from the people I've talked to online and now met in real life, particularly radical feminists on reddit and Twitter, and other parents and professionals. Everything I have written, outside of my personal story, is either just bigging up other people, or stolen ideas from other people but it's all part of my quest to get transcritical thinking out in the open. I had to learn from feminism, it was the only discourse that made sense of a transcritical perspective, but also forced some hard questions about myself and how I live my life. Encounters with feminism on my journey as GenderCriticalDad have made me realize how deep sexism goes, how it leads me to be a misogynist sometimes and how this limits me. The Radical Feminism I found teaches me that I need to reject masculinity, not as a grand gesture to the world, but in life and actions with those I care about. Not as a declaration. Not out of guilt or shame, but a hunger to be more fully human. It's not a one-off thing but a constant questioning of 'why am I behaving like this?'

Nowadays I hope I contribute something that helps drive transcritical activism. I think the existence of a GenderCriticalDad is useful, someone who can stand up and say that not all parents support trans, that there might be another discussion to be had. Of course I'm doing a huge amount of mansplaining. The GenderCriticalDad voice will get heard sometimes when women's voices are not. That recycles oppression of women but at least some transcritical thinking does get heard and I try very hard to put across views that I hope women are OK with.

Through my transcritical journey I now know other parents are in the same situation as me. It's a massive relief to know you are not alone and other parents are just ordinary, nice muddily parents like my partner and I. As a group of people working together we aim to support each other and work to make a difference in the world by dismantling myths about trans. At the same time we understand each other's fragility. We know commitment is hard when a trans identifying child can cause your world to collapse around you. We can share feelings too raw to say in public. The rage and despair of seeing your flesh and blood drift into the trans cult and turn against you is unspeakable. The joy of an ordinary moment, smiles, fresh air and sunshine and your child just being herself and not performing gender is priceless.

It is inspiring to have been invited to write this chapter. To know that at least some people think I'm not talking nonsense all the time. It's also terrifying to be a writer in this space: GenderCriticalDad has to do the right thing, there's a pressure, responsibility and accountability that goes hand in hand with transcritical activism. I'm astonished to realise GenderCriticalDad is part of an international transcritical movement now. I may lose my personal battle with my own child. I have to face that and work out how to survive with trans harm being constantly in my life and my daughter's life. But the transcritical movement and the struggle will continue and we will drive sensible discussion eventually. I need to keep faith with this belief to keep going. I cannot accept that the lies of transgender dogma will replace reality. I'm not just a hideously bigoted parent who doesn't understand transgender politics. I am a thinking parent who has learned that transcritical thinking is vital for keeping children and young people safe. And I am going to write and talk and learn about that *ad infinitum.*

References

Adams, N. (2017) *GLAAD calls for increased and accurate media coverage of transgender murders.* http://www.glaad.org/blog/glaad-calls-increased-and-accurate-media-coverage-transgender-murders

Babcock, C. (2015) *Acknowledging Transphobia for Lesbians.* https://medium.com/@swift2plunder/acknowledging-transphobia-for-lesbians-

Brunskell-Evans, H. (Ed) (2016) *The Sexualised Body & the Medical Authority of Pornography.* Cambridge Scholars

Catt, M. (undated) https://mariacatt.com / careycallahan.com

Dennis, R.J. (2017) Here's Why Misgendering Trans People Is an Act of Violence. *Everyday Feminism Magazine* http://everydayfeminism.com/2017/01/misgendering-trans-people-is-violence

—. (2017a) No, Trans Women Are NOT 'Biologically Male' *Everyday Feminism Magazine* http://everydayfeminism.com/2017/02/trans-women-not-biologically-male

Dylan-Finch, S. (2016) 130+ Examples of Cis Privilege in All Areas of Life For You To Reflect On and Address. *Everyday Feminism Magazine* http://everydayfeminism.com/2016/02/130-examples-cis-privilege

Frostrup, M. (2017) *Bringing Up Britain: Children and Gender BBC.* http://www.bbc.co.uk/programmes/b07kq5sv

Gender Wiki (undated) *Assigned Sex* http://gender.wikia.com/wiki/Assigned_Sex

Ginelle, L. (2015) *Trans Women Are Women. why do we have to keep saying this?* https://bitchmedia.org/post/trans-women-are-women-why-do-we-have-to-keep-saying-this

Glick, S. (2015) *Students condemn project vulva for 'transmisogyny'.* http://claremontindependent.com/students-condemn-project-vulva-for-transmisogyny

Godfrey, C. (2015) *How Trans Men Deal with Their Shifting Sexuality While Taking Testosterone.* https://www.vice.com/en_au/article/how-trans-men-deal-with-their-shifting-sexuality-129

Instagram (2017) https://www.instagram.com/p/BO5khIKj0JI

Jensen, R. (2016) *The End of Patriarchy: Radical Feminism for Men* Spinifex Press

—. (2017) *Getting Off: Pornography and the End of Masculinity.* http://robertwjensen.org/articles/by-topic/gender-sexuality-and-pornography/getting-off-pornography-and-the-end-of-masculinity/

Keating, S. (2107) *Can Lesbian Identity Survive the Gender Revolution?* BuzzFeeed https://www.buzzfeed.com/shannonkeating/can-lesbian-identity-survive-the-gender-revolution

Lesbian, Gay, Bisexual, Transgender Resource Centre (undated) https://uwm.edu/lgbtrc/support/gender-pronouns

Lewis, H. (2015) What the row over banning Germaine Greer is really about. *New Statesman*, 27th October 2015

Malone, L. (2015) *Transgender Suicide Attempt Rates Are Staggering.* Vocativ http://www.vocativ.com/culture/lgbt/transgender-suicide

Mulhere, K. (2015) *Inclusive Dialogues.* Inside Higher Education. https://www.insidehighered.com/news/2015/01/21/womens-college-cancels-play-saying-it-excludes-transgender-experiences

Murphy, M. (2016) 'We need to be braver.' Women challenge 'gender identity' and the silencing of feminist discourse *Feminist Current* http://www.feministcurrent.com/2016/09/27/need-braver-feminists-challenge-silencing

National LGBTQ TaskForce (2016) *Stop Trans Murders.* http://www.thetaskforce.org/current_action/stop-trans-murders/ May 3 2016

NursePath (2017) *Some Men Have VAGINAS.* https://thenursepath.blog/2017/02/10/some-men-have-vaginas

Peoples Trust Toronto (2014) *Children as Young as Nine to Be Offered Sex Change Hormones Before Puberty.* https://peoplestrusttoronto.wordpress.com/2014/05/30/children-as-young-as-nine-to-be-offered-sex-change-hormones-before-puberty

Planned Parenthood (undated) *Sexual Orientation and Gender.*
https://www.plannedparenthood.org/learn/sexual-orientation-gender

Purple Sage (undated) *Lesbian, Feminist, Gender Abolitionist.*
https://purplesagefem.wordpress.com/

Quora (undated) *What percentage of transgender women are sexually attracted to women as opposed to men, or both men and women?*
https://www.quora.com/What-percentage-of-transgender-women-are-sexually-attracted-to-women-as-opposed-to-men-or-both-men-and-women

Reilly-Cooper, R. (undated) *More Radical with Age.*
https://rebeccarc.com/about

—. (2016) *Critically Examining the Doctrine of Gender Identity.* YouTube
https://www.youtube.com

Saxby, H. (undated) The Bias of the BBC
https://notthenewsinbriefs.wordpress.com

Serano, J. (2004) *Cocky.*
https://www.juliaserano.com/drawblood.html#cocky

Strudwick, P. (2015) *This Trans Woman Kept Her Beard and Couldn't Be Happier,* Buzzfeed, https://www.buzzfeed.com/patrickstrudwick/this-transgender-woman-has-a-full-beard-and-she-couldnt-be-happier

Taking Up Too Much Space (2008) *Put the Goddamn Space in: "transwoman" "transfeminism" "transmasculine"* October 15, 2008
https://takesupspace.wordpress.com/2008/10/15/put-the-goddamn-space-in-transwoman-transfeminism-transmasculine-etc-language-politics-1

Vabvox (2015) *Erasure: the new normal for lesbians by @vabvox*
http://www.aroomofourown.org/erasure-the-new-normal-for-lesbians-by-vabvoc

Wahlquist, C. (2106 Germaine Greer tells QA her trans views were wrong – but then reinstates them. *The Guardian.* 11th April 2016

Welsh, K. (20150 Germaine Greer is a Dinosaur – powerless against a new feminist movement. *The Telegraph,* 26th October 2015

White, P. (2015) Why I no longer hate 'TERFs'. *Feminist Current.*
http://www.feministcurrent.com/2015/11/10/why-i-no-longer-hate-terfs

Wikipedia (undated) *Gender Dysphoria.*
https://en.wikipedia.org/wiki/Gender_dysphoria

Williams, S. (2014) *Got Privilege: What is Cisgender Privilege and Why Does it Matter?* Care2 http://www.care2.com/causes/got-privilege-what-is-cisgender-privilege-and-why-does-it-matter.html

YouthTransCriticalProfessionals (undated) *Professionals Thinking Critically about the Youth Transgender Narrative* https://youthtranscriticalprofessionals.org

4thWaveNow (undated) *A community of parents & friends skeptical of the "transgender child/teen" trend.* https://4thwavenow.com

Chapter Five

'Trans' Kids: LGB Adults Come Out

Josephine Bartosch

It was my first week in a new job and I was sitting in a stuffy meeting with other professionals from the third sector, we were taking turns to talk about the projects we were working on. A local organisation had recently written a report into how the NHS treats children who think of themselves as transgender. That these children really were 'trans' was a given, and that the numbers were growing was claimed as a victory for tolerance. The respective professionals all took it in turns to nod their heads gravely, and someone mentioned the high rate of suicide and self-harm amongst 'trans' teenagers. No-one could quite remember the statistic, but they knew it was awfully high and there was general agreement that we must all 'do' more. An appropriate level of shock was demonstrated and the gay chair of the LGBT group in the area grimly informed us that parents were often unsupportive of their transgender children. At this point the butch lesbian I'd been having a laugh with earlier chimed in, and said it was a 'disgrace' that parents were still telling their kids that being trans might be a phase. The LGBT group chair then continued by informing us that the kids were in the dreadful position of having to teach their parents and medical professionals from what they learnt about gender online. At this point someone asked me to pass the biscuits and the conversation moved on to a grant scheme to insulate drafty houses.

I left the meeting, called my partner and wept with frustration. In common with too many women, my partner and I both passed through our adolescence hating our bodies. When we were children the self-hatred and confusion over sexuality manifested in eating disorders and self-harm. It was no coincidence that the pages of newspapers were filled with stories about an epidemic of girls who were starving, cutting and consuming their way to the perfect body. In retrospect I can see even our most personal of choices were informed by the media landscape that surrounded us.

Thankfully no-one handed us a knife and told us cutting off hated flesh was a healthy expression of personality. Unlike in schools today, where pro-trans lobby groups have unrivalled access to schools (Awakening Clinician, 2016) there were no school visits from pro-anorexia groups to teach us that if we hated our bodies it was ok to lose a bit more weight. Social workers didn't visit to tell us our families and doctors had a duty to support us toward our perfectly imagined body. Schools did not allow us to wear clothing that would alter our shape as is the case in schools currently endorsing the wearing of binders even though a child's breathing will be compromised, lungs can be compressed and their ribs might crack (Transgender Trend, 2016). What do these changes in responses to what children and young people are saying about their bodies mean? I wanted to find a way to talk about this, particularly in relation to adolescents encountering gender confusion and discomfort with their body as they are coming out as lesbian, gay or bisexual.

This chapter will look at some 'coming-out' stories told to me by women who understood their same sex attraction before the phenomenon of transgender children hit the headlines. I have scrutinized their experiences to see what they might tell us about how best to support children and young people who don't conform to gendered expectations.

Personal responses to social pressure

My partner and I have had many conversations about how if we were coming out now it would likely be as 'transgender' because neither of us fit into the rigid category of 'feminine'. While my thirteen-year-old peers were watching *Friends,* and coating themselves with Impulse body spray I reeked of bonfire smoke and was reading *The Beano*. My partner was gazing at her baseball boots and shuffling to Indie bands. I am grateful that we grew into healthy women and found one another. Our scars have healed and we have learnt to accept, if not love, our female bodies and we still don't fit the conventional feminine mould.

It was a shock when I learnt that my Alma Mater (perhaps that should be Pater), a progressive single sex school with a focus on science, technology, engineering, and mathematics, now accepts girls who believe themselves boys. At the time of writing a case (McCormick, 2017) is progressing through the Royal Courts of Justice against a school who suggested to a child that their identifying as transgender might be a phase; it seems there are very real consequences for those who refuse to tow the accepted 'supportive' line of agreeing that any child who says they might be trans definitely is trans. I am terrified that a generation of LGB youth are being denied the chance to learn to accept themselves through gender confusion; the growing pains of adolescence are being pathologised by the pharmaceutical industry, with ill-informed liberal adults cheer-leading to demonstrate their open-minds.

Growing into a new shape is hard. Learning to navigate the often unfair and seemingly arbitrary expectations placed on our bodies is a painful process. From lessons about firm handshakes to sitting primly with legs together; understanding, and crucially being punished for transgressing, the rules can be baffling and exhausting for adolescents. These rules change over time and across different cultures, but what remains constant is that men are positioned the default. To take our places as women in today's society we have no choice but to collaborate, and it is unfair to focus on individual responses to a structural problem. Whether we shave our legs, inject toxins into our faces or have surgery, to varying degrees altering our bodies as women is expected and inescapable.

Tabloids and broadsheets alike react with predictable outrage to the behaviour of girls who ape the women in their lives in preparation for the role society has cut out for them. It was recently reported (Mackenzie, 2017) that girls as young as nine are seeking labiaplasties. Girls who don't know what a vulva is, (media reports and potential patients consistently referring their vulvas as 'vaginas') are somehow sure their own is wrong. This has been greeted with shock across the media. There is however, no corresponding righteous indignation from the press about girls who bind their breasts and aspire to double mastectomies; that 70 per cent of those referred to the Tavistock and Portman Clinic are girls who wish to be boys (Davies-Arai, 2017) passes without comment or critique.

Body modification, whatever form it takes, is a personal response to social pressure. Trying to opt out by appearing to be the other sex is yet another symptom of social malaise; it allows those oppressed by an unfair system to gain power and the feeling of autonomy over their bodies. At present, well-meaning attempts to support vulnerable people are preventing scrutiny of the social forces that underlie the desire to change sex. Silencing those who are sceptical of transgender ideologies does nothing to help those who identify as transgender, whether they are adults or children.

Feminists have long recognised that often what is presented as 'progress' in fact bolsters the status quo (Goude, 2016). The list of social changes that are apparently liberating for women is endless and yet mysteriously none have ended male violence or heralded the dawn of a brave new matriarchy. To my mind, the current popular understanding of gender identity as innate should be added to this litany of so-called 'progress' that has historically impeded the liberation of women. Belief in 'born this way' gender identity positions the inferior social position of women as inevitable and immutable. The consequences for women as a class are disturbing, but the implications for adolescents who experience same sex attraction are truly chilling.

Gender behaviour in childhood and homosexuality

In February 2017 researchers at Cambridge published a study of 4597 children exploring links between gender nonconforming behaviour in childhood and adolescent homosexuality (Gu Li, 2017). They concluded *'children who exhibit more gender non-conformity with regard to toys, playmates and activities are more likely to report more same sex and/or less other-sex attraction and behaviour'*. The authors added that their findings supported other research in suggesting *'childhood gender nonconforming behaviour is a consistent early predictor of future non-heterosexual orientations'*.

The Cambridge study is just one in a mounting body of research that suggests that 'cross sex' stereotypical behaviour and preferences are a childhood indicator of same sex attraction in adults. The same traits are identified by the NHS as evidence of being transgender. The NHS Choices website suggests the following as symptoms of a child being transgender:

> "disliking or refusing to wear clothes that are typically worn by their sex and wanting to wear clothes typically worn by the opposite sex; disliking or refusing to take part in activities and games that are typically associated with their sex, and wanting to take part in activities and games typically associated with the opposite sex; preferring to play with children of the opposite biological sex" (http://www.nhs.uk)

When the origins of these claims that such symptoms comprise 'evidence' of being transgender is collated however, it turns out that only a few established vested interest lobby groups which dominate the campaign for transitioning children and young people have been consulted (namely GIRES, Mermaids and Gendered Intelligence). From my personal experience, as further demonstrated in the interviews that follow, and indeed based on my understanding of current research, lesbian bisexual and gay (LGB) people almost invariably say they displayed behaviour in childhood that would now be wrongly taken as evidence of their being transgender if the above NHS suggestions were applied. At the time of writing I have not found policy or guidance that reflects the concerns or experience of LGB adults on these matters. I have written this chapter because I have much data to impart as will be seen in the stories of those who have contributed.

What follows are extracts from interviews with women who understood their same sex attraction before the phenomenon of transgender children hit the headlines. They vary from young women in their twenties at the time of publication to those who came out forty years ago. The experiences they describe speak of a range of conflicting feelings from comfort found in women-only space to the social pressures each of the women had to contend with. I am not claiming these interviewees are representative of the LGB community but I think the power of the voices of a small group of women sharing their experiences offers intelligence and insight to a debate which is otherwise being smothered by the biased voices of equally unrepresentative transadults.

Ally's story

Ally is a 27 year old barrister living in London. She married her female partner last year. It was at the age of fourteen when Ally says she was first honest with herself about her feelings for other women and she told her friendship circle about these at fifteen. Ally contrasts the accepting attitude of her friends at her progressive girls' school to those of her Catholic parents, whose reaction she described as 'dreadful'. After being out as a 'gay' for a year she tried to please her family by having boyfriends. She explained that she dated *'harmless, kind boys, but boys I had no feelings for. It wasn't until I recovered (from an eating disorder), that I began to re-engage with and embrace my true feelings for women'*. Reflecting on these relationships, Ally described them as 'really harmful'. Opposite sex relationships are a recurring motif in coming out stories; same sex attraction doesn't free those who experience it from internalising the prejudices that surround us all. Enduring unwanted relationships demonstrates how powerful shame and the desire to please are.

Ally considered that she might have understood her identity differently if transgender identities had been as prominent as they are now saying:

> I think I would have been trans in some way. I wouldn't go so far as to say I would have thought I was male, as stereotypically, I always presented fairly "femme" as lesbians go (ugh). However, as a teenager who was going through huge problems with body image/eating, I know that I would have sought solace in say, non-binaryism. It would have helped me to escape my womanhood. … I came out at fourteen or fifteen

> but for several years after this, once my eating disorder kicked in, I had no feelings for anything or anyone

She also thinks she would have been subject to physical harm had she interpreted her identity as transgender:

> I think it would have been very harmful to me as a vulnerable teenager to have been more aware of transgenderism. I am sure I would have worn a binder in my efforts to suppress my body. It's quite sad really, because once you start suppressing your body, you suppress your sexuality.

Binding breasts can result in punctured lungs and permanent spinal damage (Peitzmeier, 2017) and yet it is not recognised in the UK as a form of self-harm. The practice of breast binding has become so normalised UK schools have been advised to modify Physical Education lessons to accommodate girls who can't breathe fully due to wearing binders (Sandeman, 2016). In our allegedly enlightened times breast ironing, foot-binding and corsetry are widely recognised as forms of violence against women, but binding of developing adolescent girls bodies is supported by the very organisations that should centre the welfare of children. The parallels between traditional methods of self-harm and expression of transgender identity amongst adolescents cries out for further investigation. Frustratingly, with the academy ever more in the grip of 'progressive' group-think this seems increasingly unlikely.

Snow's story

Snow, a lesbian in her early twenties from the Midlands says she first recognised herself to be a lesbian at the age of fourteen. Her family were not supportive and she felt 'forced back into the closet' until she was twenty-one because of the absence of *'support from anyone around me and lack of lesbian role models'*. Snow raises a serious concern about the impact of transgender movement on young people trying to understand their sexuality. She herself struggled to find support online, and noted *'most 'lesbian' blogs that offer 'support' are run by bi women who tell young questioning lesbians that they have to be open to sex with penises or they're transphobic'*. She continued:

> if I was, say, a fourteen year old questioning lesbian two years ago, as opposed to a twenty-one year old, then I feel it would be very easy to be misled into thinking I was an awful person for my sexuality and to be led in to trying to change in a different way. Basically, homophobia caused me to suppress my sexuality and date men, and what the Transactivists

spew is just repackaged homophobia from liberal audiences rather than conservatives.

Snow's account refers to the line increasingly taken by mainstream 'feminist' and LGBT online resources. For example, *Everyday Feminism* has become one of the most popular feminist digital media sites in the world boasting a readership of 4.5 million monthly visitors. Riley J Dennis, a key contributor to the site whose YouTube videos regularly score hundreds of thousands of hits, argues that *'genital preferences are transphobic'* (Dennis, 2017).When transgender ideology is followed to its logical conclusion sexual orientation in any form ceases to exist as 'gender identity' is not deemed related to the physical sex of a body. This idea is most commonly weaponised against lesbians who refuse to consider transwomen as sexual partners. Transactivists rail against what they term 'the cotton ceiling'; the 'cotton ceiling' they argue they are excluded from penetrating is that of women's underwear.

Reflecting on the impact of transgender ideologies on lesbian identity, Snow recalled a painful conversation with a lesbian friend who identifies as 'queer':

> I remember her asking me 'would you ever sleep with a transwoman?' and I had to dart around the question, fearful that she would hate or reject me if she knew that I, a lesbian like her, wasn't willing to sleep with even post-op transwomen.

A sense of loss at a proud lesbian identity is articulated in more depth by others interviewed, as is frustration at the narrow confines of femininity. Similarly to Ally, Snow considers that she *'would've identified as non-binary, if that was a thing back in 2007'*. She explained:

> I've seen a few posts online about how 'non-binary' is this generation's answer to a lack of a 'gender-bending' teenage subculture existing. I believe that's true. I can't pretend that teenage me wouldn't have embraced the fashionable aspect of being 'non-binary'.

Non-binary identities are increasingly adopted by those seeking to free themselves of gender stereotypes. Ironically, insisting on a separate category for those who want to opt out of gender all together reifies a binary that demands the rest of us must be content to accept our sexed labels. Arguably such insistence is an unhelpful, albeit perhaps understandable, attempt to identify out of the stereotypes that hurt us all. Non-binaryism also sits directly at odds with the popular notion of gender as a spectrum; if we are all somewhere between masculinity and femininity then by definition we are all 'non-binary'. Nonetheless, the appeal to young people of having a claim to being like others is understandable. Snow describes how in secondary school she struggled to fit in:

> I often wished I was a boy, because boys could be loud and funny and have weird senses of humour. My few friends were male nerds, and the popular girls often laughed at their jokes, while they looked down on me. I detested how the girls would giggle at the boys' antics, and be clean and coy and care about makeup, and so I detested girls in general. I declared I was 'not like other girls', and non-binary is basically the modern version of that. I didn't realise at the time that I didn't hate girls but I hated how girls were supposed to be. I hated the feminine gender role, and hated how I had a lot of trouble conforming to it. I believe non-binary girls see themselves as fully realised human beings rather than pretty dolls, but they fail to realise, like I did as a kid, that no girl truly identifies with being non-human.

The division of women into competing factions, and the internalised misogyny of those who don't feel they fit, makes young lesbians easy prey for an ideology that allows them to opt out of the 'girl role'. Moreover, violence against women in pornography is currently an ordinary part of most adolescents' sex education (Crabbe, 2016). When becoming a woman, let alone a woman who loves women, is so fraught with internal body hatred and external threat, perhaps it isn't surprising that increasing numbers are rejecting lesbianism and opting to present as transgender or non-binary.

That both Snow and Ally endured unwanted relationships to satisfy their parents shows how entrenched homophobia is. The label and accompanying medical treatments of the transgender identity are perhaps more comforting than accepting one's sexuality; being transgender locates the problem in the mutable body rather than in a rigid society or errant self. A transgender individual can control their appearance to fit in with societal expectations of 'normal' behaviour; someone who is same-sex attracted will always by definition be 'abnormal'. Parents and children who might never have considered their own homophobia can find a medical solution that will help their same-sex attracted child conform to homophobic values. Transgender identities offer an appealing solution that may allow some families to side-step discomfort about same sex attraction and the accompanying awkward topic of sexual desire.

Jen's story

Jen describes herself as coming from a *'poor area in the North of England'* where *'there was no representation of gender non-conforming women anywhere'*. From childhood to adulthood Jen has been deliberately misread as male; first from the age of eight as a form of playground bullying when she was 'constantly called 'a boy'' and then at university where she was told she was transgender by her peers. Jen explains how she navigated her identity at university and the 'huge resistance' she encountered for rejecting the 'queer' label:

> At University I was often understood (assumed) to be Trans, asked if I was Trans fairly consistently (mirroring the "are you a boy or a girl?" I got at school or as street harassment) and even told I was Trans, thanks to the kindly Queer feminist queers at Bar Wotever (where you can be 'whatever' bar someone who rejects self-defined categories or identities). I get all that could have acted as a form of seduction, but I was definitely not seduced.

That Jen had the self-awareness and presence of mind to refuse such crudely imposed labels is impressive. She continued by outlining how the transgender narrative would have been attractive to her when she was younger and more vulnerable:

> I imagine the homophobic abuse I experienced, not for being in a relationship with another girl, but for not looking like a girl should (why 'transphobia' is most often homophobia in practice), could've been eclipsed by saying *"well, actually I am a boy, so fuck off"*. But then I'm aware that women aren't allowed to encroach on male society, no Transmen get to [encroach on male society] so it actually might have been no real help. When I talk to de-transitioned women they do say the need to escape the glare of the male gaze and homophobia towards them was a real pole of attraction for transition and I can relate to that.

Reflecting on the support groups she encountered at University Jen commented:

> When I think back to the Women's Society at University it is the case many of its former prominent members are now Transmen. All of those who transitioned were /are lesbians. I didn't employ much thought into this at the time, but noticed a consistent trend looking back. I actually no longer know of more than handful of gay women under 30 nowadays. There is a marked absence. So whilst most Transmen stay within the lesbian community it has added to [the lesbian community's] ever-

diminishing status and populace. I hope that's reversible through some sort of renewal. If we look at what's happening, from San Francisco to London, there are no lesbian bars or spaces anymore. It's a lot to reverse.

It certainly seems lesbianism has an image problem; perhaps it conjures up images of dental dams and the sensible shoes of the seventies that don't translate to the Instagram era. Interestingly, the younger women in these interviews all rejected the word lesbian when they came out, with Ally commenting that herself and her friend would; *'refuse to use the word 'lesbian' as we thought it was quite porny. This was in about 2006. Perhaps the word lesbian had already gone out of style by then'*. This chimes with my experience. I remember my partner quipping that the term 'lesbian' sounds like a disease, and until recently she was one of many women who opt for the male descriptor 'gay' or the catch-all 'queer'. As some of these contributors opine, there are the 'sexy' and deeply unconvincing lesbians of male pornographic fantasy, but where are real life lesbian role models? It seems lesbian communities have been fractured by the inclusion of transgender people and eclipsed in language and reality by the more fashionable queer identities.

Jen's reflections lead in to perhaps the most divisive and hotly debated topic for feminists and lesbians which focuses on who is accepted into women-only space. How you feel about this matter hinges on whether one accepts self-definition or female biology and socialisation as the marker of womanhood. For transwomen who consider themselves lesbians being a part of women only-space is of course a validation of their identity and many seek these groups out.

In the UK, the Transgender Inquiry Report (Women and Equalities Committee 2015, 2016) recommended that The Equality Act of 2010 be updated to include 'gender identity' as a protected characteristic. This will force women to accept anyone who identifies as such into their space, putting a legal nail in the social coffin. The parallel debate in the US has focussed upon access of transgender people to their preferred toilet, the implications of self-identification for sex-segregated changing rooms, refuges, prisons, hospital wards, smear tests and rape crisis centres are seldom mentioned. On the upside transmen will finally be free to enjoy a round of golf at The Royal Burgess Golfing Society.

Esme's story

Esme is 43; she came out as lesbian at 30 having previously lived with a man for eight years from the age of eighteen. She described her relationship with a male partner as 'a form of escapism'. In her words Esme wanted 'to be normal' and ignored her feelings for women until she explored them during therapy in her mid-twenties. She joined the local LGB group, (before the 'T' was added) and met new friends and her first girlfriend; previously she hadn't known any other lesbians and being involved with the group helped her to feel part of a community.

In common with Ally, who described 'taking comfort' in portrayals of lesbians in popular culture, Esme said:

> Looking back before I realised I was a lesbian I did have a particular fascination with lesbian characters and storylines (not many of them back then in mid -late 1990s). I watched the Ellen 'coming out' episodes and the first lesbian kiss on TV with Anna Friel on Brookside. Seeing lesbians on TV was actually a massive part of my journey to realising I was one. I didn't know any lesbians in real life and my views of lesbians were very stereotypical.

The increased visibility of lesbians in the mainstream media over the past ten years is to be applauded, and clearly it helps women understand their sexuality. Regrettably it seems producers feel they have now largely *done* lesbian storylines. The new addition of 'transgender' and 'non-binary' to the range of possible identities is ripe with sexy new appeal. At the time of writing, it is impossible to imagine a programme about a lesbian child, and yet programmes such as 'I am Jazz' a reality show about a child who identifies as transgender are streamed into the U.K. from the U.S. television. For Esme, finding a mirror of her desires on screen helped her to realise her identity. Those same desires are now too frequently framed as evidence of being transgender; the impact and appeal of this to children and young people questioning their sexuality should not be underestimated.

The medium of choice for younger people is now online viewing, where they are able to watch content produced by their peers. At the time of writing, a YouTube search of 'trans coming out' yields 2,440,000 results. The narratives of teenage YouTubers explaining their transgender identities are identikit; their identification as transgender is always entirely explained in terms of a preference for the stereotypical clothes, activities and interests of the other sex, peppered with self-loathing.

One might hope that professional journalists and producers would notice the privilege being afforded to transgender children and be concerned about equality of representation and presentation of balanced material, but it seems transgender teens make a great story. Frustratingly it is not just the gutter press that bulges with such stories; from the BBC (*I Am Leo*) to National Geographic (*Gender Revolution*), respected outlets are uncritically promoting the message that children's bodies should be changed to match stereotypes about sexed behaviour.

Esme continued her reflections with a heartfelt explanation of how crucially important she found women-only space when she was coming out and how she needed these spaces as she battled to address *'internal misogyny and lesbophobia'*:

> For me being with and sharing experiences with women is an essential part of lesbianism. I would not have been comfortable if there was any hint of having to accept trans-lesbians. I was also in a fragile place with a history of childhood sexual abuse and had been hospitalised for mental health issues and so I would not have attended [women-only or lesbian spaces] if men were there. This time in my life was about coming to terms with my own femaleness and female sexuality.

Ashamed of being a lesbian and a woman, Esme said she had desperately wanted to belong somewhere as a child/teenager. She thought it 'very likely' that she would have identified as transgender had she not had therapy to help her explore her feelings. Esme detailed her nonconforming behaviour prior to coming out:

> I did not identify as a lesbian until I was 30 and did not consider it part of my sexuality until my mid-twenties. From a young child I was gender non-conforming. I did not feel comfortable as a girl. I did not like girly things. I wanted to be a boy. I valued boy things over girl things. I used to get mistaken as a boy. I wanted boy muscles and to be strong like a boy. I had short hair. I liked making stuff, getting dirty, played with my brothers action men not dolls. I hated pink. I hated all the girl stereotypes. I chose metal work and woodwork at school instead of cooking. I studied science at University and actively looked for a male dominated career – engineering. I didn't want to do a girly job. I felt self-conscious to be female; ashamed to female.

Today Esme proudly declares she is 'glad to be a woman' with 'male-stereotypical' interests and hobbies. She realises with some trepidation that even as a young adult becoming a man would have been appealing as it wasn't until beginning therapy that she 'came to accept and value being a woman'. Fifteen years ago therapy helped Esme understand the dysmorphia she felt about her body, without automatically seizing upon that dysphoria as an indication that she must begin a process leading to taking testosterone and having surgery to remove her breasts. However, earlier this year the Chief Executive of the UK Council for Psychotherapy issued a statement of 'solidarity against conversion therapy' which now places young people experiencing gender dysphoria on a direct trajectory to chemical and surgical intervention. The statement of 'solidarity against conversion therapy' is based on contributions for the chairs of the Royal College of GPs, British Psychoanalytic Council, British Association for Counselling and Psychotherapy and the President of the British Psychological Society. It declares:

> We have always been clear that sexual orientation and gender identities are not mental health disorders. Any therapy that claims to change these is not only unethical but it's also potentially harmful. (British Psychoanalytic Council 2017)

Esme's experience raises considerable cause for concern over the abovementioned position. Arguably, based on her experience, the statement of 'solidarity against conversion therapy' is poorly conceived modern-day virtue-signalling revealing approaches to sexual orientation which clearly should be challenged to allow the valid practice of questioning gender identity to support a wide range of underlying causes of body dysmorphia.

It must be remembered that there is no biological basis to transgender identities; theories of brain sex have largely been disproved. The nebulous concept of 'gender identity' that we must all accept for the theory to be valid has yet to proven. That medical (NHS, n.d.), legal (Women and Equalities Committee, 2016) and social changes have been established in the absence of any evidence points to domination of a powerful and vocal trans-activist lobby. The credentials of this lobby are far from straightforward. The affirmation approach (paraphrased as *'if a child thinks they might be transgender, they must be affirmed as definitely transgender'*) championed by the World Professional Association for Transgender Health (WPATH) (Anon., n.d.) has been accepted by the medical establishment in the UK yet WPATH are reticent about identifying their sponsors; there is evidence to suggest sponsors include huge pharmaceutical and health companies, including Glaxo-Smithkline, Bristol-Meyers-Squibb and Johnson & Johnson (Anon., n.d.). Jennifer Pritzker, who was James until August 2013, recently joined the 48 women in the Forbes list of the 400 Richest Americans. Pritzker is a transwoman philanthropist, funding numerous transgender-focussed organisations, from the Transgender Military Service Initiative to the Gender & Sex Development Program at Lurie Children's Hospital. Those sceptical of the transgender ideology cannot hope to compete with this level of funding.

Last year when I wrote to my MP with concerns on the topic of gender affirmation during therapy he sent me back a standard response informing me that he was proud his government no longer deem being transgender to be a mental illness. I am left pondering what other condition with no readily definable cause in the body legitimates the removal of healthy tissue and the lifelong administration of powerful drugs without questions asked and raises only a standard self-satisfied reply to expressed concerns.

Given the likely numbers of lesbian and gay people who have had irreversible medical treatments to affirm a straight identity, the 'conversation therapy' charge levelled at open-minded counsellors today seems bitterly ironic. Had Esme had asked for advice now that the statement of 'solidarity against conversion therapy' prevails, it is highly likely that her therapist would have no option other than to affirm Esme's body dysmorphia as evidence of a transgender identity. This issue is discussed further in relation to teenagers nowadays in chapters by GenderCriticalDad and Moore (this volume).

As I was collecting Esme's story it was reported that Angelina Jolie and Brad Pitt's daughter, Shiloh identifies as a boy (Eglash, 2017) and is due to start hormone treatment. In 2010 evidence for Shiloh's transgender identity was offered by Jolie as follows: *'She likes to dress like a boy. She wants to be a boy. So we had to cut her hair. She likes to wear boys' everything. She thinks she's one of the brothers'*. The reaction of Shiloh's celebrity parents has been heralded as supportive and their daughter is now referred to by male pronouns across the gossip pages of glossy magazines. Shiloh is 11 years old at the time of writing. Hormone treatment will prevent her experience of growing into a woman at the same pace as her peers, compromise her fertility and 'literally' block crucial life experience key to beginning to understand her sexuality.

Louise's story

Louise is 51. She was born into a working class community in the North East of England. Louise has lived with the woman to whom she now is civil-partnered for 25 years. In her own words, Louise realised the 'irrefutable fact that I was a lesbian called 'me'' at the age of 19, when she was disowned by her family. She explained 'it was the realisation of what being a girl was that set me on my path, and, for me, the right path' and continued:

> I was 5 when I was made to realise that I was failing the expectations placed on little girls. I was active, and physical, mischievous, strong, funny. I was curious and fearless, brave. Dolls bored me, prams turned into tanks or go-karts. I excelled at sport, football in particular. I was clever and one of those children who absorbed information. I was quick

to see how the world worked. It seemed to me that the words 'just a girl' and 'girls don't do this/that' were too common. And 'NOT ALLOWED' pertained more to my sex than the other!

The messages that boys/men were the pinnacle of human evolution and us girls/women were a sort of afterthought; 'not quite as good as' went against everything I was feeling. My body and brain worked just as well. I was confused, curious and quite angry about the unfairness of it. Women and girls were everywhere but seeing them doing, being or achieving anything were mostly ignored, rendered invisible or twisted into something completely different. I knew I couldn't be unique, it didn't make sense that other girls wouldn't be like me. Which lion cub comes out of its mother's den being told 'you're just a lioness, nothing to fear here?'

I started to look for women and girls doing things other than pleasing 'people', mainly men, anywhere and everywhere. So, at an early age I was exploring my femaleness.'

It was at fourteen or fifteen years of age that it began to dawn on Louise that her interest in other girls had a sexual dimension, and at seventeen she told her mother she was a lesbian. Louise describes being 'ostracised emotionally' by her family who had 'no empathy with anything outside the realms of normal'. Between the ages of fifteen and eighteen Louise began to consider whether she wanted to be a man. She explained her "isolated, unsupported, ill advised 'self' struggled with the lack of affirming 'blue print' to living'. On recognising the options open to men but denied to her Louise considered whether it would be easier if she were a man. The idea upset her greatly:

> I was beyond bereft. I did not want to be male. The young girl wanted to be the best girl I could be; physically and mentally. I had become increasingly assured that my sexuality was 100% lesbian, although I had tried to do the boy/girl teen thing, I hated it, I had been excellent at passing as 'straight girl' but had never been close to hetero sex.

Louise explained that coming out for her 'involved in the perceived rejection of everything' that she had previously understood to be 'normal'. It was at 19 when she was a student that she fully embraced being a lesbian. Becoming politicised about Clause 28 offered an external focus that galvanised her identity. Interestingly, the other women interviewed do not explicitly mention an interest in politics. The post-modern approach that has emerged as dominant since Louise came out in the 1980s favours identities over ideologies and an internal focus on the self rather than a critical analysis of the structures by which the self is defined. Transgender identities fit neatly within this mould, that a change is needed is a given, though the concept of 'gender' that was once seen as emanating from a sexist society, has been turned inward as an identity. As Louise put it:

> My demeanour, my clothes, my hairstyles, my character traits, my interests and certainly my sexuality confounds so many 'feminine' stereotypes as prescribed by society and how women should behave. Yet, I am a woman. Gender is a performance, a game. My sex is unchangeable.
>
> When I was 'coming out' I was told, in general, 'you want to be a man' because I wanted to be intimate with women. This is the misogyny/homophobia of the mainstream because to envisage a positive reality which does not involve men is the most subversive act. ...My real power as a lesbian whether I am having sex or not is my culture, history, my sense of self awareness and the knowledge I hold, affirming my existence. I don't need medication, surgery, or laws to know it. My sexuality is lesbian.
>
> I have spent many decades searching for myself in literature, art, music, history, politics, science, philosophy...women are there doing, and being, inventing, thinking. We have been extraordinary. In every aspect of life, we have been there, but too often ignored. If that rich tapestry of femaleness had been celebrated equally I would have realised that I was a lesbian when I was about six or seven years old.

Lesbian voices and the intransigence of transgender ideology

On the surface the stories of lesbian women I have interviewed for this chapter are different. What links them is resistance to sexist stereotypes that dominate our lives as women and resistance to a heteronormative society. All of the women who contributed to the chapter proudly embrace their lesbianism and nonconformity, though each of them struggled to come out. Painfully present in both the coming out stories of lesbians in these pages, and the adolescents of today who identify as transgender, is the fear of growing into adult bodies that are bound by stereotypes. There are striking parallels between eating disorders and self-harm trends in previous decades and the current prevalence of gender dysphoria. All of these issues disproportionately affect girls going through adolescence. In addition as discussed across this book, children who consider they are transgender are not only likely to grow into LGB adults, they are also more likely to be on the autistic spectrum or to be gifted. A common denominator underlying their identification as transgender is a feeling of 'not fitting in'. What is chilling about the phenomenon of childhood transgenderism is that unlike phenomenon that potentially harm children and young people, no sensible discussion of possible harms is allowed and policy and practice increasingly dictate that transgender identification must be cheered on *regardless of known harms* by adults who should have a responsibility to urge caution. Happy and safe outcomes for the women who contributed to this chapter would likely be very different had they struggled to understand their sexuality in the context of transgender ideology that currently cannot be questioned.

Younger generations of women largely accept the self-definition model of womanhood; this is fiercely policed and those who question an individual's self-definition face being ostracized, as both Jen and Snow atone. When this is compared to the politicising and affirming experience of university life as recalled by Louise it is clear that the tyranny of identity politics has fractured what was once a women-led movement of collective struggle. My observations of the LGBT community mirror this; today's Pride marches are a hollow celebration of ever more niche identities and a marketing opportunity for rainbow-clad corporate sponsors rather than a political protest. There is a palpable sense of loss in these stories; the women interviewed who drew strength from sharing an experience with others know that important spaces are gone.

As Ally commented *'if I were in a lesbian group now and there was a trans-identified male present, I would find it very, very difficult to stay a part of that group'*. It is not surprising that so few young lesbians recognise themselves as such when the communities left to guide them through the coming out process are dying. As Jen observes, increasing numbers of younger women are choosing to become transmen. Having a pseudo-biological reason why you don't fit is comforting; it seems being a lesbian is just a bit *gay*.

From Caitlyn Jenner in the US to India Willoughby in the UK, it is photogenic older transwomen who tend to be those chosen to pose in the media spotlight, and the majority of them lived as straight men prior to their transition. Those who exist in their shadow are young transmen. To my mind the transition of girls who don't conform to sex-role stereotypes is a new front of the war on women, with the bodies and needs of children struggling to become women, being sacrificed to validate the identities of a group of adult men. That this is dressed in progressive politics makes it all the more insidious.

Professionals with a duty to protect children are effectively hailing the sterilisation of lesbian, bisexual and gay adolescents as evidence of social progress. All of the women who contributed their stories are clear they would have found some temporary solace in transgender identities. Whether they are representative of today's young people who identify as transgender or not, in this chapter there are testimonies from five women who today would be denied the chance to come to terms with their female bodies, and indeed to become mothers. There is a shameful history of patriarchal medical practices being played out on the bodies of those who don't conform. It is my belief that the medicalisation of children who don't fit gender stereotypes will be remembered alongside the clitorectomies performed on women and girls deemed to be 'hysterical' and those labelled 'Sapphists' in the nineteenth century.

We owe it to children to be adults who are not afraid to speak out; protection of children from known harm must come before our own desire to seem progressive. Furthermore, professionals must stop colluding in convenient lies to boost their careers and find the personal integrity to think and speak critically about the ideologies behind gender identity. It is sexism and homophobia that must change, not children's bodies. No child has the 'wrong' body, they have their own body and their body is their own.

References

Awakening Clinician (2016) *Awakening Clinician, UK: What do we think we are talking about?* Youth Gender Professionals https://youthtranscriticalprofessionals.org/2016/04/24/awakening-clinician-uk-what-do-we-think-we-are-talking-about/

Anon., n.d. http://www.wpath.org/site

Anon., n.d. *Gender Trender.* https://gendertrender.files.wordpress.com/2015/05/wpath-2003-corporate-funders.jpg

British Psychoanalytic Council (2015) *UK Organisations Unite Against Conversion Therapy - Solidarity with like-minded organisations in the USA* https://www.bpc.org.uk/news/uk-organisations-unite-against-conversion-therapy-solidarity-minded-organisations-usa_Accessed 06 07 2017

Crabbe, M (2016) *Making Violence Sexy: Pornography, Young People and Sexuality.* Pornography and Harms to Children and Young People Symposium, February 2016, Sydney Australia

Davies-Arai, S. (2017) *From Adult Males To Teenage Girls – The Movement From Etiology To Ideology.* https://www.TransgenderTrend.com/from-adult-males-to-teenage-girls-the-movement-from-ctiology-to-ideology/ Accessed 05 07 2017

Dennis, R. J. (2017) *Are Genital Preferences Transphobic?* https://www.youtube.com

Eglash, J. (2017) *http://www.inquisitr.com/4188070/angelina-jolie-brad-pitts-daughter-shiloh-jolie-pitt-sports-new-short-hairstyle-amid-transgender-rumors* http://www.inquisitr.com/4188070/angelina-jolie-brad-pitts-daughter-shiloh-jolie-pitt-sports-new-short-hairstyle-amid-transgender-rumors/ Accessed 05 07 2017

Goude, G. (2106) *Gender Is Not An Identity; It Is A Tool of Patriarchy.* @gencritgreen Gendercriticalgreens.wordpress.com

Gu Li, K. (2017) Childhood Gender-Typed Behavior and Adolescent Sexual Orientation: A Longitudinal Population-Based Study. *Developmental Psychology*

Mackenzie, J. (2017) *Vagina surgery 'sought by girls as young as nine.* BBC Victoria Derbyshire programme. http://www.bbc.co.uk/news/health-40410459 Accessed 05 07 2017

McCormick, J. P. (2017) *Pink News* http://www.pinknews.co.uk/2017/07/04/teen-sues-private-school-after-being-told-being-trans-was-a-phase/amp/

NHS Choices (2009) *My Trans Daughter* http://www.nhs.uk/Livewell/Transhealth/Pages/Transrealstorymother.aspx Accessed 14 February 2017

NHS n.d. *Gender Dysphoria Symptoms* http://www.nhs.uk/Conditions/Gender-dysphoria/Pages/Symptoms.aspx Accessed 05 07 2017

NHS n.d. https://www.england.nhs.uk/wp-content/uploads/2017/04/ gender-development-service-children-adolescents.pdf

Peitzmeier S. (2017) Health impact of chest binding among transgender adults: a community-engaged, cross-sectional study. *Cult Health Sex,* pp. 64-75

Sandeman, G., 30. (2016) Struggling To Breathe. Councils tell schools to give transgender pupils 'extra PE breaks' because of chest-binding practice https://www.thesun.co.uk/news/1527158/councils-tell-schools-to-give-transgender-pupils-extra-pe-breaks-because-of-chest-binding-practice/, *The Sun*

Transgender Trend (2016) *Breast Binders In UK Schools* *https://www.Transgender Trend.com/breast-binders-in-uk-schools/*

Women and Equalities Committee (2015) *Transgender Equality Report* https://publications.parliament.uk/pa/cm201516/cmselect/cmwomeq/390/39002.htm

Women and Equalities Committee (2016) *Transgender Equality Inquiry* https://www.parliament.uk/business/committees/committees-a-z/commons-select/women-and-equalities-committee/inquiries/parliament-2015/transgender-equality/

Chapter Six

The Language of the Psyche: Symptoms as Symbols

Lisa Marchiano

The Glass Delusion

From the 15th through the 17th centuries, one of the most common psychiatric afflictions was called "the glass delusion". Sufferers believed they were made of glass and must be treated with extreme care lest their limbs shatter. One of the first cases was King Charles VI of France, who forbade people to touch him and swathed himself in protective blankets (Inglis-Arkell, 2014).

This mental health disorder may have gotten a celebrity start with the French king, but it spread. For approximately 200 years, people all over Europe developed symptoms of the glass delusion; many of its victims were from the wealthy and educated classes. By the 1600s the glass delusion was a cultural phenomenon and the most noteworthy mental illness of the times. Cervantes wrote a short novel about it (Inglis-Arkell, 2014). Rene Descartes mentioned it (Inglis-Arkell, 2014). And then it disappeared. By the 1800s there were few reported cases (Inglis-Arkell, 2014). The cultural unconscious had found other images and symbols through which to express psychic pain.

The dictionary defines "delusion" as "an idiosyncratic belief or impression maintained despite being contradicted by reality or rational argument" (Stevenson, 2010). It comes from the Latin word *deludere,* which means to mock. *Ludere* is Latin for "to play," and the prefix *de* gives the word a pejorative meaning. To play is to inhabit the space between what is fixed and what is false. A delusion then, is play that has become stuck. Play has degraded into dangerous fixity. To avoid falling into delusion, we must find a way to inhabit the *in between* space of authentic play, the realm of imagination, creativity, ritual, dreams, shamanism—and psychoanalysis.

The great British psychoanalyst D. W. Winnicott attached enormous importance to play, and felt that psychological health involved being able to relate flexibly to the inner world of fantasy as well as the outer world of consensual reality (Winnicott, 2005). We need access to both. Winnicott coined the term "transitional space" to describe the in between territory in which play unfolds. The transitional space between external and internal worlds can be a place of encounter with new aspects of self, unthought truths, and creative solutions. "It is in playing and only in playing that the individual child or adult is able to be creative and to use the whole personality, and it is only in being creative that the individual discovers the self" (Winnicott 2005, 72-73). When we lose contact with the realm of *in between*, we lose access to the transformative space where change and healing happen.

When a client expresses a desire to change something in his or her external world, I hold it in Winnicott's transitional space. I often find myself saying: "I don't know what your feelings mean, but I do know they are important". I attempt to acknowledge the person's emotional truth while holding open the myriad ways it might be lived in the external world. My words express my belief that the voice of the soul finds ways of speaking that are surprising, weird, inconvenient, improbable, and disruptive. But to live a life awakened to individual meaning, we must take psyche's voice seriously.

To take something seriously, however, does not mean taking it literally. There is a space *in between* where metaphor proliferates, and curiosity is cultivated. If we cannot access the *in between*, we either reject expressions of soul as mere delusion, or we take such expressions concretely. The symbolic content that the psyche would have us look at becomes concretized and flattened, or brushed aside as "nothing but". Either way, we forfeit the ability to see a larger psychic and symbolic meaning. The work of attending to soul means trying to carefully inhabit that middle, *in between* space of the symbolic realm.

In listening for the voice of the psyche, we must listen into the *in between*, and neither dismiss our soul's messages nor construe them too concretely. Tuning into the poetic voice of the psyche can help us understand the recent surge in young people taking on non-traditional gender identities as a demand of a generation to have their struggles taken seriously in a world that has largely forgotten how to find this in between space. "There is no illness," Jung wrote, "that is not at the same time an unsuccessful attempt at a cure" (Jung 1966, 46). I argue that adopting a transgender identity may be just such an attempt at a cure on the part of young people struggling to find a meaningful initiation into adulthood. Transition comes from the Latin word "trans" which means to go across, to go beyond. In our culture of out-of-control materialism, is it any wonder that young people are desperate to go beyond? Identifying as transgender is an attempt to transcend the limits of biology to live out an *inner* reality. Feelings associated with gender take on the importance of personal revelation, compensating for a culture in which the literal and logical is so overvalued and soul is often denied. Ironically, in the case of medical transition, the compelling inner experience becomes hypostatized, metaphor made flesh. The young person falls into the sin of concretization even as he or she tries to break free from it.

In this chapter, I will explore transgender identities among adolescents as a symbolic communication of psychic conflicts that are a normal part of the painful and often frightening passage to adulthood. In doing so, I will draw upon my clinical work with parents of transgender teens. The analysis presented here is my own thinking, informed by my work and training as a Jungian psychoanalyst. Jung taught us that our unconscious has important things to tell us, and that it does so in the symbolic language of myth, dream, and ritual (1970). Only by staying open to the psyche's strange symbolic tongue can we hear what it wants to tell us. To respond to the sudden rise in transgender self-diagnoses among young people in a manner that will enable personal and collective growth and transformation, we must be willing to engage the symbolic dimension of the symptom.

Liminal & Literal

Winnicott's transitional space overlaps a great deal with the anthropological concept of liminality, a term coined by the French ethnographer Arnold van Gennep (1960). In his 1906 book *The Rites of Passage*, van Gennep wrote about initiation rituals around the world. He noted that such rites always follow a common pattern: separation, transition or liminality, and reincorporation. In the first stage, the initiate takes part in symbolic acts that separate him from his former self and his former place in his tribe. He cuts away the person he has been, preparing to enter the liminal phase (van Gennep, 1960).

Liminal comes from the Latin word for threshold. It is a passage from one state to another, a crossing over marked by ambiguity and disorientation. Van Gennep also referred to this part of the rite as transition; things at this stage are in a state of flux. According to van

Gennep, in this stage, social hierarchies are collapsed or dissolved. Norms are reversed, as one thing becomes its opposite. The middle liminal stage is where the main transformations of initiation occur.

Van Gennep described tribal rites characterized by a middle period of liminality, when monsters become incarnate, people die and are reborn, and the initiate is disoriented and unsure. Liminal experiences—such as religious rites, dreams, creative expression, and psychoanalysis—require things to be *both and*. We relate to the fantastic images that come up from the unconscious with a double stance—one from each side of the threshold—and allow that they express a legitimate psychological truth, even while we do not expect them to conform to objective consensual reality. *Harry Potter* author J. K. Rowling captures the essence of what it means for something to be psychologically true in dialogue between the young wizard and the elder Dumbledore. When the pair meet in liminal space after Dumbledore's death, Harry asks whether the experience is real, or just happening in his head. "Of course it is happening inside your head, Harry, but why on earth should that mean that it is not real?" replies Dumbledore (Rowling, 2007, 723).

Examples of engaging psychological truths seriously but not literally are easy to find. An indigenous shaman turns into an eagle at night, picks up the sick person he is to heal, and flies with him on his back to the Milky Way. Sticks are inserted into their bodies. They fly back, the shaman sucks the sticks out of his patient, and cures him (Bosnak, 1996). Such liminal experiences are now being rediscovered by young people, who share them through social media. Nineteen-year-old John from Knoxville identifies as a fox:

> "I started getting odd dreams where I would change physically into a fox, and they were very realistic—honestly. And after a while, in real life, it felt quite real, like I actually had a tail, I actually had ears, I actually had paws. At first it was one of those things that I freaked out over, and then after a while it was like ah... I'm just gonna play with my tail for a minute." Every so often, John says he gets mental shifts: "I could just be at home, and all of a sudden, click, the fox part of me just kind of comes out for a while, and then it just goes" (Roberts 2015).

When John's experience of fox-ness is held as a liminal experience, it has all the richness and healing potential of the shaman's eagle flight. If understood as inner experience, it can lead him to greater appreciation of the spaciousness of soul. If, however, we make the mistake of understanding this experience concretely, it loses its symbolic potential for healing and veers alarmingly into delusion. Instead of leading us to curiosity about our inner life and an integration of our own mysterious and archetypal fox-like qualities, the experience becomes inappropriately transplanted to the realm of the literal, where it can lead not to wholeness, but to increased isolation and suffering. John's experience would then be reduced to pathology.

Dennis Avner was an American of Lakota and Huron heritage (Hall, 2012). At ten, he was given the name "Stalking Cat" by a medicine man. Later, a chief exhorted him to "follow the ways of the tiger". Avner identified with his totem animal and appears to have understood this instruction concretely, for in adulthood he began to modify his body. Sometimes without anesthesia, Avner subjected himself to 14 surgeries to make himself look more feline. His septum was altered to flatten his nose, his teeth were capped and filed into points, silicone pads were implanted in his cheeks, and his upper lip was split. In 2012, at the age of 54, Avner was found dead in his apartment of apparent suicide (Hall, 2012).

Although causes can only be assumed, Avner's search for transformation through surgery represents a collapse of the liminal, imaginal engagement of tiger-ness that might have transformed his life from the inside. When liminal space collapses, as it apparently did for Avner, we lose access to the renewing source of psychic life. Avner's quest for concrete realization of his tiger-ness apparently failed to lead to psychological health. So too we must be circumspect about a young person's desire to concretize a threshold experience via medical transition. Concretizing feelings by medicalized body alteration is likely to mean that the subtle messages from the unconscious are not being engaged symbolically.

Symbolic Understanding

The middle, liminal space is the realm of the symbolic. According to Jung, a symbol does not have a fixed meaning but points beyond itself to a larger content that can never be fully encompassed by image or word 1975. It is the best expression for something unknown and essentially unknowable (1975). Understanding something symbolically is never a reductive process but one that adds layers of meaning. The image becomes larger and more spacious, getting both more specific and precise and less so at the same time.

When I was a child, my family owned a set of encyclopaedias, and I used to love to sit and flip through the volumes. One of my favourite entries was the one for the human body. The illustration included an inset of the different systems—circulatory, digestive, muscular, skeletal, etc.—

each printed on a separate sheet of clear plastic, so that they could be layered over each other, giving a sense of how the systems interrelated. Holding a symptom, feeling, or image in a symbolic fashion is somewhat like these illustrative overlays. Each layer adds something, perhaps obscuring something else, but not replacing it. Each level of meaning expands the experience of the original so that it is always more than the sum of its parts.

A teen "comes out" as transgender. If we understand this revelation concretely, we will see a girl trapped in a male body or vice versa, a cognitive construction that wasn't even possible until recent advances in medical technology. We are then held fast to this one-dimensional, limited understanding, and as with Dennis Avner's facial surgery, a literal understanding may seek external world realization. A symbolic perspective allows us to find companionship and encouragement in the universal human experience of feeling estranged from ourselves and our bodies. We are no longer fixated on those aspects of our experience that separate us and mark us as different, but find instead reassurance and connection with all who live and who have gone before us.

Taking symptoms concretely means that we may miss the meaning behind how our suffering has expressed itself. We focus on the wrapping, not the contents. This is always a possibility in the case of psychological symptoms. With body dysmorphia, for example, cosmetic surgery is contraindicated, for follow-up data show that the patient's obsessive dissatisfaction with one body part doesn't disappear after the "flaw" is corrected with surgery. Rather, it migrates to some other part of the body, which then becomes the new focus of intense dislike. The real suffering has not been addressed through surgery.

Tyler, a young transman, had a phalloplasty leaving him with a large scar on his arm. He posted a video entitled "I Hate My Arm":

> I worked so hard for this body, and now I'm not ashamed of the parts I was before. I don't experience dysphoria, I don't hate my body. Now it's all about my arm. I can go out shirtless, I can go out naked if I want, but my arm would be covered, no matter what. I want to start forcing myself out of sweatshirts and long sleeved shirts and forcing myself to go out and show my arm, but any time I think about it I just get sick to my stomach 'cause I'm so afraid (Tylerjvine 2016).

This is what Jung meant when he said the "neurosis is always a substitute for legitimate suffering" (Jung 1969, 75). When we focus on the outer manifestation of the trouble, we are avoiding a genuine encounter with suffering. If we cannot encounter our suffering, we cannot hope to discover the kernel of transformative potential within it.

In the case of a transgender teen, I argue that the cure is not to fix the symptoms in objective reality, where the treatment dictated is a medicalized, concretized changing of names, hairstyles, and bodily appearance. Altering appearance is often a futile effort to capture the elusive intricacies of the psyche in fixed, physical form. That the "cure" for transgenderism has been reduced to commodified medical procedures focused on external appearance indicates that we may be addressing a soul problem in the superficial realm of persona, as the pathos of Dennis Avner's history attests.

Does the psyche ever want the concrete thing? The body of a tiger or the opposite sex? Could it be that a symbolic experience of our inner reality might also need to be lived out concretely? Possibly—but let's be wary. Without a willingness to explore, to be curious, or even mistaken, a rigid definition of the problem usually indicates an ego-driven stance. When someone comes into treatment and is certain that the only solution to the presenting problem is something in the outer world—a new job, a new partner, a new body—in my experience, it is almost always the case that the person is avoiding the deeper message conveyed by the pain.

The current cultural prescription for how to work with transgender youth does not allow for doubt. Transgender advocates aver certainty about innate gender: that we definitively know our own "authentic self," and that physical transition is the right course toward this authenticity. They exhort parents that full affirmation of a child's self-diagnosed identity is crucial for that child's well-being (Brill, 2016). Part of the appeal of these beliefs is that they offer such a certain way to understand the ordinary tragedy of passing over the threshold to adulthood, along with a clear prescription to fix it. Let's reclaim the psychic space *in between* and engage the mysteries of symbol to help us understand the recent surge in young people taking on non-traditional identities. Such an approach can open up multiple ways of relating to a child's identity exploration and help us to divine the underlying issues, as described in the following case example.

Mikayla/Mitch*

Vicky is a middle-aged woman in my practice. She had been in treatment with me for some time before her daughter Mikayla began to struggle with gender. The following is a summary of her experience dealing with her daughter's transgender identity in the context of the work she and I did together to understand Mikayla's experience within a developmental framework that considered the symbolic aspect of adolescent identity exploration. For clarity's sake, I will refer to Mikayla by masculine pronouns and name when recounting the part of the story during which she identified as transgender.

Mikayla is the only child of Vicky and Tom, who divorced when Mikayla was six. After the divorce, Vicky went through a period of depression. Tom travelled much of the year, and was in Mikayla's life only sporadically. Most of the time, Mikayla lived with her mother. Vicky states that Mikayla's childhood was mostly unremarkable. She fell in love with horses as a little girl, and rode at a nearby stable for many years. Vicky also remembers that Mikayla and a neighbourhood friend used to like to pretend that they were dancers in a music video, and would spend hours making up their own dances in the garage. Mikayla was academically advanced, and loved to read. Science fiction was always a favourite genre. Throughout grade school, she tended to have one or two friends with whom she was very close. Her mother described her as intense, quiet and somewhat anxious. Mikayla was nine years old when her cat died. Mikayla stopped eating for several days and refused to go to school for over a week due to grief and a paralyzing fear that the same fate would befall her.

When Mikayla was thirteen, her father relocated overseas for work. Though he tried to reassure her by promising fun summers in Europe, Mikayla was devastated. She recognized, as her father did not, that their relationship would become more difficult to sustain than ever. Around the same time, an older boy cornered her backstage during a school play rehearsal and made lewd and threatening remarks while friends of his laughed nearby. Mikayla had felt the boy was a friend and was deeply shaken by this incident. Her mother reports that Mikayla started wearing baggy, oversized sweatshirts after this. She stopped doing the play or singing in the choir, activities she had previously enjoyed. Mikayla became withdrawn and unreachable, and spent long hours in her room on her computer. Vicky admits that she was aware that Mikayla was probably on her computer late into the night, but felt that separating her from her friends on social media would only make her more alone and unhappy.

A few months after the backstage incident Mikayla gave her mother a letter stating that she was transgender. To Vicky, the wording of the letter seemed formulaic, unlike Mikayla's own style. She is pretty sure that Mikayla copied a template letter from an online site. The letter stated Mikayla's desire to be addressed as Mitch and referred to as "he". The letter also included a plea for hormone blockers, along with a vaguely worded threat: "If I am not able to interrupt the wrong puberty my body is starting to go through I am afraid for my future".

At first, Vicky was shocked and saddened. Vicky had never seen any behavior in her child that would lead her to believe she was struggling with gender. In addition, the idea that her daughter might really be her "son" made her grieve for the child she had always known and loved. But she was worried about her child, and she wanted to be as supportive as possible. Worried about Mikayla's recent tendency toward isolation and depression, Vicky quickly conceded on the matter of pronouns, name, and haircut. She even bought the child she was now calling Mitch a breast binder. However, she stated that she needed more time to consider before she would agree to Mitch taking medication.

Now in the 9th grade, Mitch began presenting as male at school. He was readily accepted in a peer group that was predominantly other natal females who identified as "transmasc," gender fluid, nonbinary, or some other designation. At first, Vicky was pleased to see Mitch gaining confidence and having friends after being socially isolated. But she also felt uneasy. "When they came over to the house or I drove them somewhere, gender issues were all they ever spoke about," she said. "It seemed to me there was something unhealthy about their preoccupation with all of this. I could see Mitch was getting swept along by them. I just hoped it was for the best."

After a few months, Vicky's hope was waning. The more time Mitch spent presenting as a transman, the unhappier he seemed. He became obsessed with passing as male. His academic performance worsened. He became further isolated from anything not trans related. His preoccupation was ruminative, leading him to focus on perceived slights or threats. When a family friend accidentally "misgendered" him by using female pronouns at a dinner gathering, Mitch became sullen and quietly enraged. He left the table and retreated to his room. When Vicky eventually forced her way into his room, she found that he had cut the word "die" into his arm with superficial scratches; he confessed contemplating taking a bottle of pills. Mitch was hospitalized briefly for suicidal ideation. Gender issues were not a focus in the hospital, and Mitch had a break from the Internet and obsessing about identity. Vicky reported that he seemed a little better once he was home. The hospitalization also gave Vicky a chance to take a brief break from her constant worry and think; she made some changes when Mitch came home. First, she made a point of not talking about gender issues.

Engaging Mitch on this topic seemed to make him more spun up and anxious, and led to conflict no matter how carefully supportive Vicky attempted to be. It seemed that when the two of them discussed anything having to do with Mitch's gender, Mitch began the conversation from a standpoint of being certain that his mother would not understand. Not surprisingly, he usually had this expectation met, and the talk ended with Mitch more withdrawn and anxious. So Vicky quietly avoided the subject. But she did not avoid Mitch.

She made a point of spending more time together, doing things he had always enjoyed. They took a weekly creek walk as they had often done when Mitch was younger. She started to ask Mitch to walk the dog with her in the evenings, and he often came. Vicky told me she had decided it didn't matter whether the two of them talked when they were together. She didn't try to fill the space. But they were together, and most of the time after one of these brief trips around the block with the dog, things felt a little easier, a little less strained, even if neither of them spoke a word. Vicky started suggesting the two of them go to a movie every Friday. She was surprised when Mitch almost always said yes, often even turning down invitations to spend time with friends. Vicky and Mitch were developing a connected routine that was fun and pleasant for them both.

Vicky began to see that Mitch's trans identification was in part an effort to separate from her, while at the same time asking for more care, attention, and connection from her. When Vicky responded to the latter request by spending time with Mitch without bringing up gender, there was de-escalation in household tension. If Mitch did bring up gender, Vicky attempted to address the issue in a neutral manner. When it came time to go to a family wedding and Mitch stated that he wanted to wear a tuxedo, Vicky didn't make a big deal out of it. "It's just clothing," she said. Occasionally, Mitch would try to bait her with provocative statements. For example, when he was feeling particularly distressed, he would blame Vicky, saying that he was miserable because she didn't believe he was truly trans. At these times, Vicky attempted to validate Mitch's feelings of distress without getting sucked into an argument about transgenderism.

Mitch's discharge plan from the hospital had included a recommendation that he start attending a weekly support group for trans-identified teens at a local center. In the weeks after Mitch's return from the hospital, Vicky noticed a pattern. The support group met on Wednesday evenings. Mitch would return from the support group sullen, withdrawn, and self-righteously argumentative. Thursdays were often difficult days as well. However, within a day or two, Mitch started to settle down again and be more relaxed in his mother's company. By Saturday or Sunday, Mitch would appear less anxious and depressed, and more able to engage in helping around the house, or doing his schoolwork. This would be the case until Wednesday evening, when the cycle would begin again. Of course, there were sometimes angry outbursts and times when Mitch withdrew even during the "good" part of the week. Vicky noticed these often occurred around something that made Mitch anxious, such as final exams. Though Mitch's rants would focus on Vicky's lack of support for his trans identity, Vicky began to suspect that these episodes were mostly about Mitch's fear of failure, which stemmed from his perfectionism.

Throughout, Mitch continued to find satisfaction in sketching, an activity that had always been a favourite. Even at his most depressed, he would draw for hours and always signed up for an art class in school. Mitch's art teachers nominated him for a summer art program in Italy for talented high school students. Mitch's first reaction was ambivalent. He was thrilled by his teachers' confidence in him, but felt anxious about traveling alone and navigating identity issues overseas. He would have to live in a dorm, for example, and the dorms were grouped by sex. Vicky saw this as an opportunity for Mitch to have a significantly broadening experience. She gently encouraged the idea. Mitch was accepted to the program and agreed to go. With minimal discussion, Mitch agreed to be housed in the girls' dorm, though his presentation when traveling continued to be androgynous. The program rules stipulated that phone calls were allowed only once per week. The program's website, however, posted photographs from time to time, and Vicky had glimpses of Mitch engaged in art projects or attending museums with other participants. She was delighted and relieved to hear excitement in Mitch's voice during their weekly phone calls. Mitch was swept away by all of it: new friends, the ambience of Italy, and the professional art instruction.

Mitch's absence gave Vicky a chance to step back and look at the bigger picture—something that she and I were able to do in our work together. We had often discussed the possibility that the trauma Mitch had experienced backstage may have made him feel frightened to be perceived as female. We also discussed the probability that constant exposure through social media and his peers may have convinced him that identifying as transgender made sense for him. But Vicky had another interesting insight:

> "I am realizing that I never gave Mitch his own space around the separation and divorce. I never intended to ask him to take on my stuff, or turn him against his dad. But when I got depressed, it really affected

him. I thought I was just being open, but I can see now that telling him about my own struggles was too much for him."

Movingly, Vicky had come to see the ways in which she and her child had become psychologically fused. She speculated—and I agreed—that Mitch's transgenderism was perhaps in part an effort to separate from her and develop a unique identity, while simultaneously signalling distress and anger at Vicky for her post-divorce collapse.

When Vicky met Mitch at the airport six weeks later, his hair had started to grow out, and he was sporting new clothes purchased in Italy. The two of them hugged and cried, and then went straight to one of Mitch's favourite restaurants. When Vicky referred to him by Mitch, he corrected her. "You can go back to calling me Mikayla and using feminine pronouns. I don't think I'm a typical girl, but I'm not a boy either. Maybe I really am a lesbian. I don't know. But I do need to change schools. Please don't make me go back to Central." Vicky was able to make a last-minute school change happen, and in September Mikayla started 10th grade as a girl. She continued to wear her hair short, and dressed mostly in baggy sweatshirts and jeans. At times, she could still become overwhelmed by anxiety. But she was less prone to dark moods. She was often happy and playful, and Vicky reported that she felt as though her daughter had come back to her, even as Mikayla started to look toward going to college and leaving home.

Vicky and I came to understand that, for Mikayla, adopting a transgender identity seemed to be both a plunge into depths of dark emotions and an attempt to avoid growing up. Binding her breasts, cutting her hair and begging for hormone blockers were efforts to deny her maturing female body. Her focus on being trans was also a way to avoid developmental challenges by displacing them onto gender, and her mother and school personnel avoided stressing her due to perceived fragility around gender. Like a bird feigning a broken wing to draw a predator away from a nest, Mikayla used gender confusion to draw attention away from developmental demands she was unready to face. Mikayla's trip overseas served as the positive initiation into adult life she may have been trying to find in her trans identification. It allowed her to have needed, healthy separation from the narrow confines of home and school. Her weeks abroad connected her with a larger world and allowed her to experience an expanded sense of self and imagine a new future. Mikayla's trans period served both as a defense against unbearable present reality, and provided something transcendent to bridge the impasse. As with all psychic products, Mikayla's transgender identity may also prefigure in symbolic language the direction in which her soul needs to grow. As

Mikayla continues to mature she can claim her "masculine" traits, becoming fearless, boisterous, loud, opinionated, strong, and confident.

Initiation

Throughout human history, cultures have developed rites of passage to help young people cross the threshold into adulthood, and from this we can surmise that adolescents have an ancient need to undergo initiation. If there are no elders present who can lead them through a meaningful initiation, teens unconsciously seek other ways. As youth approach adulthood, their developmental need to discover meaning and purpose draws them into the fires of life. They look for intense and even dangerous situations in which to test themselves, and they seek a tribe to which they can belong. Identifying as transgender may in some cases be an attempt to self-initiate, to slip the bounds of banal ordinariness and seek meaning and transcendence.

All initiations have at their core a death and rebirth experience as has been documented by anthropologists (Eliade, 1975, van Gennep, 1960). Initiates are often considered dead during the liminal/transitional period of the rite so that they may be resurrected in adult form. Often, they receive a new name upon completing their initiation. Many trans-identified children and their parents view transition as the death of an old self and the rebirth of someone new. Nine-year-old Ash, for example, thinks of the male part of herself as an older brother "that died or fell off a cliff" (France, 2016). Indeed, a trans person's birth name is universally referred to as a "dead name" (Talusan, 2015).

In indigenous initiations, the initiate sometimes undergoes a painful scarification or mutilation of his body in a "procedure of collective differentiation" that connects him forever onward with other initiated adults and conveys his new status in visual form (van Gennep, 1960, 74). The ritualized hair and clothing styles, body piercings, tattoos, and even surgeries involved in social and medical transition mark the non-binary or trans teen as part of a tribe. The young person has achieved a new status indicated by physical difference. He or she is no longer a child. By claiming a transgender identity, the young person may be attempting to separate herself from her childhood and mark an initiation into adulthood.
However, for initiations to do their work, they must engage the unconscious and be negotiated in the liminal realm, for the passage from childhood to adulthood is an existential crisis at the heart of which lies the question "who am I?" The initiate must die to childhood. This is an intensely painful and frightening process made more so today because

many young people must undergo adolescent initiation unaccompanied by formal rites. The collective experience, elders, and the language of ritual that has historically made meaning of this momentous transition is mostly absent in our culture. Today, the developmental crisis of adolescence is no longer contained by collective structures designed to help the young person successfully negotiate this perilous psychological crossing.

Mythologist Michael Meade has noted, "literalism is the great spell that binds and blinds the modern world" (Meade 2006, 122). If elders can't help adolescents hold their quest symbolically, but collude in seeing their exploration as literal, there is a risk that teens will become stuck in this transition phase. Then the initiation will be incomplete. To help young people hold their transition into adulthood symbolically, we must be committed to the importance of their experience without shrinking it into its literal manifestation. I contend that we must see *beyond* the symptom to the meaning behind it and be prepared to look more deeply at what is getting expressed individually and culturally.

Initiations require ordeals, and these are always painful and frightening. As initiating elders, part of our role will be to witness our children's suffering and discern when it is senseless and ought to be stopped, and when it is the sort the broadens and deepens, awakening the young person to what is hidden in his soul. If it is the latter, we must avoid the temptation to "fix" the suffering by addressing it superficially. As elders, we understand that this painful trial has deep significance in the symbolic realm. We hold open the liminal, transitional space so that the young person can retain access to it, and so can experience her initiatory suffering as that which helps her to hear the story that came with her into the world. The way of initiation for women has always entailed going down into dark earth. The earliest myths of feminine initiation—from Innana in Sumeria to Persephone in ancient Greece—depict it as a fearful journey into the depths. During such a journey, the world of childhood is left behind and innocence is sacrificed. With her mother's help, Mikayla experienced her descent as transformative, and returned from the depths a maturing woman.

Teens for whom gender exploration is a descent to the underworld of depression, anxiety, and rumination need us to meet their ordeal with the spaciousness of symbolic understanding rather than the rigidness of certainty. The word "metaphor" comes from a Greek word meaning "to carry over." As we try to make sense of a teen's descent, the poetic language of metaphor can help carry us over the gulf of understanding and break the spell of literalism, allowing the ordeal to become an experience that transforms.

The case of Mikayla/Mitch is a fictionalized composite of many stories I have heard from parents.

References

Bosnak, R. (1996) *Tracks in the Wilderness of Dreaming: exploring interior landscape through practical dreamwork.* New York: Delacorte Press

Brill, S. (2016) *The Transgender Teen: a handbook for parents and professionals supporting transgender and non-binary teens.* San Francisco, CA: Cleis Press

Eliade, M. (1975) *Rites and Symbols of Initiation.* New York: Harper & Row

France, L. (2016) "Inside Britain's only transgender clinic for children." *The Times*, November 5, 2016 http://www.thetimes.co.uk/

Hall, J. (2017) *The Independent.* November 14, 2012. Accessed January 08, 2017 http://www.independent.co.uk/news/people/news/stalking-cat-daniel-avner-found-dead-in-apparent-suicide-after-years-of-body-modification-to-look-8316569.html

Inglis-Arkell, E. (2014) *"The "Glass Delusion" Was The Most Popular Madness of the Middle Ages."* Io9. September 18, 2014. Accessed February 24, 2017. http://io9.gizmodo.com/the-glass-delusion-was-the-most-popular-madness-of-th-1636228483

Jung, C. G. (1966) *The Collected Works of C. G. Jung. The spirit in man, art, and literature.* Edited by Herbert Read, Michael Fordham, and Gerhard Adler. Translated by R. F. C. Hull. New York, NY: Bollingen Foundation

—. (1969) *The Collected Works of C.G. Jung. Psychology and religion: West and East.* Translated by R. F. C. Hull. Edited by Herbert Read, Michael Fordham, and Gerhard Adler. 2nd ed. Princeton, NJ: Princeton University Press

—. (1970) *The Collected Works of C. G. Jung. Symbols of Transformation.* Translated by R. F. C. Hull. Edited by Herbert Read, Michael Fordham, and Gerhard Adler. 2nd ed. Princeton, NJ: Princeton University Press

—. (1975) *The Collected Works of C.G. Jung. The Structure and Dynamics of the Psyche.* Translated by R. F. C. Hull. Edited by Herbert Read, Michael Fordham, and Gerhard Adler. Princeton, NJ: Princeton University Press

Meade, M. (2006) *The Water of Life: initiation and the tempering of the soul.* Seattle: Greenfire Press

Roberts, A. (2015) "*Otherkin Are People Too; They Just Identify as Nonhuman.*" Vice. July 16, 2015. Accessed January 08, 2017. http://www.vice.com/en_ca/read/from-dragons-to-foxes-the-otherkin-community-believes-you-can-be-whatever-you-want-to-be

Rowling, J. K., and Mary GrandPre (2007) *Harry Potter and the Deathly Hallows. (Harry Potter series, year 7.).* New York: Arthur A. Levine Books/Scholastic Inc

Stevenson, A. (2010) *Oxford Dictionary of English.* Oxford: Oxford University Press

Talusan, M.R. (2015) "*What 'Deadnaming' Means, and why you shouldn't do it to Caitlyn Jenner.*" Fusion. June 4, 2015. Accessed February 26, 2017. http://fusion.net/story/144324/what-deadnaming-means-and-why-you-shouldnt-do-it-to-caitlyn-jenner/

Tylerjvine (2016) "*I Hate My Arm*" YouTube. September 26, 2016. Accessed January 08, 2017. https://www.youtube.com/watch?v=vseH5D8e3A8

Van Gennep, A. (1960) *The Rites of Passage.* Chicago: University of Chicago Press

Winnicott, D.W. (2005) *Playing and Reality.* New York, NY: Routledge

Chapter Seven

The Body Factory: Twentieth Century Stories of Sex Change

Susan Matthews

The twentieth century was fascinated with the meaning of sex and gender, fascinated too with the possibilities of bodily alteration. This chapter argues that by reading stories from the past we can not only trace fears that the transgender narrative now seeks to conceal but also identify what is new about current transgender discourse. Imaginative writers both echo and predict the innovations of science. For instance, the twentieth century was the century of synthetic hormones, "from the earliest days of endocrinology in the 1890s through the first heyday of HRT in the 1960s" (Watkins, 2007). Sex hormones were studied intensively in the 1920s with the "scientific and commercial development of pharmaceutical oestrogen in the 1930s" (Watkins, 2007). These new medical discoveries may find an echo Virginia Woolf's 1928 *Orlando*, the story of a young man who lives from the time of Shakespeare until Woolf's present and who becomes a woman along the way. Woolf's fantastical tale does not just echo medical discoveries but uses fiction to challenge gender norms and to reject essentialism: "The change of sex, though it altered their future, did nothing whatever to alter their identity". It suggests the underlying androgyny of human identity: "In every human being a vacillation from one sex to the other takes place, and often it is only the clothes that keep the male or female likeness, while underneath the sex is the very opposite of what it is above." Orlando becomes a woman when the possibilities open to women change through history. In a key scene, her multiple identities pass through her mind:

> For she had a great variety of selves to call upon, far more than we have been able to find room for, since a biography is considered complete if it

merely accounts for sex or seven selves, whereas a person may well have as many as a thousand. Choosing then, only those selves we have found room for, Orlando may now have called on [...]the boy who saw the poet; the boy who handed the Queen the bowl of rose water; or she may have called upon the young man who fell in love with Sasha; or upon the Courtier; or upon the Ambassador; or upon the Soldier; or upon the Traveller; or she may have wanted the woman to come to her; the Gipsy; the Fine Lady; the Hermit; the girl in love with life; the Patroness of Letters.

Compare the real-life Margaret Anne Bulkley who in 1808 wrote "Was I not a girl I would be a Soldier!" before adopting a male disguise and practicing as a Dr James Barry (Du Preez and Dronfield, 2016). The twentieth century marked a growing tendency to view experience "in a medical framework where the medical view is seen as the authoritative, if not hegemonic, view" (Preves, 2002). The first novel to describe a physical sex change may be Gore Vidal's 1968 *Myra Breckinridge*, published soon after the Johns Hopkins gender identity clinic began surgical gender reassignment. Twentieth century fictions show that the story of "transgender" is a recent invention that the "authentic self" realized through "gender affirmation" is, historically, as new as the technologies that make it possible.

A Brief History of Gender

According to the sexologist John Money "It is impossible to write about the social and political history of the second half of the twentieth without reference to the concept of gender" (Money and Ehrhardt,1996). Money (who we will be meeting again later in the chapter) liked to claim that he had invented the concept – indeed a recent sympathetic account of his career is called *The Man Who Invented Gender* (Goldie, 2014). Certainly the word took on new meanings in the second half of the twentieth century and is now central to how we think about ourselves. Yet as Deborah Cameron points out, many of the key texts of second wave feminism including Simone de Beauvoir's 1949 *The Second Sex* make their arguments without using the term (Cameron, 2016). The OED (in an entry revised in 2011) gives 1947 as the first use of "gender" to mean "The state of being male or female as expressed by social or cultural distinctions and differences, rather than biological ones," the "socialized obverse of sex". As a word for a grammatical feature of language, "gender" dates from 1390 but up until the twentieth century it could also function as a neutral term for "A class of things or beings distinguished by having certain characteristics in common." While the "masculine" or "feminine gender" grouped together men or women, it was equally possible to refer, as Shakespeare did in *Othello,* to "one gender of hearbes" or as Robert Bage does in 1784, to the "patriotic gender." In 1847, there were even genders of shawls: the "rectangular shape is preferred for all articles of this gender, except for the India shawl" (OED Online, 2016).

The word "gender" takes on its familiar opposition to "sex" in the second half of the twentieth century in the wake of changes in the meaning of "sex" and "sexuality" (Smith, 2000). When Coleridge coined the word "bisexual" in 1825, referring to "The very old Tradition of the Homo Androgynous, i.e. that the original Man...was bi-sexual," he did not mean that the original man was "sexually attracted to individuals of both sexes" (a meaning that first appears in 1914) but that an innate androgyny is natural – an assumption that, as we have seen, exists in Woolf's *Orlando* (Jackson, 2010). Coleridge suggested that all human beings contain within them both gendered identities or, as we might now say, everyone is gender non-binary. For when Coleridge was writing, the word "sex" referred to a category of human beings defined by their bodily difference (women were "the sex" or the "fair sex" in the eighteenth century). As "sex" came to refer to erotic acts rather than bodies (a meaning first recorded by the OED in 1900), this left a gap for a word to describe men or women as a group, a gap filled by the word "gender". There is no doubt, then, that the terms within which we understand our identities have changed and that our current understanding of gender is specific to our own time and culture.

Crossing the divide

Attempts by historians of sexuality to rediscover a lost history of homosexuality have struggled with the changing language of sexuality (Foucault, 1978; Norton, 1992; Hobson, 2000). Understandings of sexuality have changed over time, just as the words we use to define them have too. Historians of transgender are confronted by similar problems. Because the medical technologies of sex change are a twentieth century invention, trans history has sometimes corralled transvestite as well as lesbian and gay experience from the past. Modern taxonomies are applied to past lives: Margaret Anne Bulkley, aka Dr James Barry has recently been described as "gender-fluid" (Pulver, 2008). Transvestism is now retrospectively reclassified as transgender history: Susan Stryker, for instance, describes Hirschfeld's 1910 *The Transvestites* as "the first book length treatment of the transgender phenomenon" (Stryker, 2008). But contemporary transgender ideology is distinct from earlier attempts to cross the divide of sex or of gender.

Contemporary transgender narratives understand and narrate body modification in new ways. Take for instance, removal of the testicles ("orchiectomy" or "orchidectomy"). In 2017, "gender surgery" or orchiectomy on a seventeen-year-old can be represented as "what happens to women just trying to be at peace with themselves and their bodies" (Duffy, 2017). An inner truth of gender, a kind of gendered soul, is imagined as made manifest by "gender affirmation" surgery. Contrast Balzac's 1830 story "Sarrasine" in which a sculptor falls in love with what he takes to be the most beautiful woman he has ever seen. But the opera singer, La Zambinella, is revealed as a *castrato*, a boy castrated before puberty to preserve his unbroken voice. The singer does not see himself as a woman: "What if I were not a woman?", he warns. Gender clinicians as late as the 1990s were fascinated by the history of castration which they did not understand as "gender affirmation": Russell W Reid's presentation to the GENDYS conference in 1994 described the role of castration in the Russian Skoptic sect which persisted for two hundred years from the eighteenth century. Reid (1994) explained that "the genitals, particularly the testes, were considered the organs of lust, wickedness, impurity and evil" which must be removed in order to enter the Kingdom of God. Reid drew his account from a 1988 paper by sexologist John Money, who wrote in another context: "I suffered from the guilt of being male [...] I wore the mark of man's vile sexuality" – that is the penis and testicles (Colapinto, 2013). Late twentieth century stories of sex change often represent a feminist attack on man's "vile sexuality". In Angela Carter's 1977 novel, *Passion of New Eve,* Evelyn is forcibly castrated by a female cult in punishment for his treatment of women. Carter identifies the cultural idealization of femininity as the dark obverse of misogyny: in this novel the silent movie star Tristessa St.Ange who represents the perfect woman (as in Balzac's "Sarrasine") turns out to be a transsexual.

The Body Factory

The radically new belief that you can be born in the wrong body allows contemporary transgender ideology to assert that a trans identity is innate. I'm going to argue that two late twentieth century stories of sex change allow us to capture the shift in gender ideology that makes such a belief possible.

The story that finally emerges from Iain Banks' 1984 novel *The Wasp Factory* is that a young girl was attacked by the family dog while her mother was in labour with her younger brother. Although the father pulled the dog away and the girl's genitals were not fundamentally damaged, the father brought his daughter up to believe that she was a boy castrated by the dog. He makes a wax model of infant testicles which he keeps in a jar in his office in case proof should be needed and surreptitiously laces his daughter's food with male hormones. Believing herself to be a castrated male she displays an over compensatory masculinity expressed in the motiveless murder of two children. The novel ends as "Frank" discovers the deception and realizes that he is a woman. Frank's unreliable narration has tricked the reader into sharing Frank's erroneous belief that he is male.

Although my second story is not fiction it has entered modern myth. David Reimer's story has been told many times: in medical papers and books by John Money and others and in John Colapinto's 2000 popular non-fiction account *As Nature Made Him: The Boy that was Raised a Girl* (Money and Ehrhardt, 1996; Colapinto, 1997, Eugenedes, 2002). Reimer's story was also told in a series of BBC documentaries beginning with "The First Question" in 1980 which Banks conceivably might have seen. Reimer was born in 1966 as Bruce, the identical twin brother of Brian, but was accidentally castrated at the age of nine months in a medical mistake during circumcision. The parents contacted gender identity specialist John Money who recommended bringing up the boy as a girl and the infant had further surgery to remove his testicles. At twelve the girl was given female hormones. But by the age of fourteen she had become depressed and extracted the truth from her parents. She transitioned to living as a male, choosing male hormones and genital reconstruction.

Reimer's story has taken on an extraordinary cultural power: Natalie Angier (1997) wrote that "the case [...] has the force of allegory"- though as Judith Butler (2004) pointed out, no one seems to agree on what the allegory means. Reimer's story has been used as evidence for two conflicting theories of gender identity. In a series of publications, John Money used the case to prove his theory of psychosexual neutrality, the idea that gender identity is "postnatal and learned," a theory that was cited by Kate Millett (1970). Following the protocol, he had established for the treatment of intersex babies, Money believed that sex could be safely reassigned within an eighteen month window after birth. He described how:

> [a]t the time of surgery, when we saw the parents in person for the first time in the psychohormonal research unit at Johns Hopkins, we gave them advice and counselling on the future prognosis and management of

their new daughter, based on experience with similar reassignments in hermaphroditic babies. In particular, they were given confidence that their child can be expected to differentiate a female gender identity, in agreement with her sex of rearing (Money and Ehrhardt, 1996).

Precisely because Reimer was not intersex and had an identical twin brother, Money saw the success of the gender reassignment as proof of his theory. The case is said to have reassured transgender pioneer Virginia Prince in her decision to undergo surgery (Colapinto, 2000). After the revelation in 1997 that the experiment had been a failure, it was used to support a new model of gender identity: "that a sense of being male or female is innate, immune to the interventions of doctors, therapists and parents" (Angier, 1997). As such, Reimer's life is now used to evidence the idea of gender identity as an inner sense of self and trans activists distance themselves from Money's work.

John Money saw himself as a story teller, mapping a new world of gender identity and sexual behaviour: "I frequently find myself toying with concepts and working out potential hypotheses," he explained. "It is like playing a game of science fiction" (cited in Colapinto, 2000). It is this culture of experiment and punishment that Banks (1984) explores in *The Wasp Factory*: Frank's "father saw [the dog attack] as an ideal opportunity for a little experiment, and a way of lessening – perhaps removing entirely – the influence of the female around him as I grew up." Frank grows up in a predominantly male setting, a Scottish island cut off from the mainland at high tide which carries echoes of the island of *Lord of the Flies*. His father uses the child to get revenge for rejection and betrayal, acting out an adult agenda. Frank of course cannot remember the scene described by his father of the dog's attack but relays it to the reader in a disturbing account in which birth (offstage) is linked to castration: "My mother was heaving and grunting, pushing and breathing, an hour or so away from producing, and attended by both Mrs Clamp and my father, when all three […] heard frenzied barking and one high, awful scream." The fake primal scene inserts itself into Frank's consciousness, emblematizing the destructive nature of women.

Reversing the gender dynamic of the Reimer case, Banks's dark fantasy suggests how a belief (in this case that Frank is a castrated male) can lead a child into an alienated relationship with their body. Determined to act out a passable imitation of masculinity, Frank hits the local pub with his friend Jamie: "I had this horrible vision of my body being made up almost completely of two equal-sized compartments, one holding piss and the other undigested beer, whisky, crisps, dry-roasted peanuts, spit, snot, bile and one or two bits of fish and potatoes". His body fragments: "I seemed to have a separate brain for each limb, but they'd all broken off diplomatic relations." Frank is troubled by his inability to take part in ritualistic masculine pissing games:

> You can score points for the number of ceramic divisions you can move the butt over (with extra for actually getting it down the hole and extra for doing it from the far end of the gutter from the hole), for the amount of destruction caused – apparently it's very hard to get the little black cone at the burned end to disintegrate – and, over the course of the evening, the number of fag-ends so dispatched [...] but it is not for me, thanks to cruel fate.

This story is the product of a culture that still assumes gender identity is defined by rearing. By contrast, Colapinto (2000) (who assumes that gender identity is innate) reports that Reimer resisted culturally enforced gender, revealing that Brenda's "stubborn insistence on standing" to urinate "created a housekeeping nightmare" for her mother.

Banks paints a nuanced picture of the relationship of individual to social beliefs. Frank's father is an anarchist rebel, a hippie who home educates his children on an island. Frank refers to "my literal cutting off from society's mainland." For a time the father dresses his older brother as a girl. But his twisted treatment of his children is also a dark shadow of social forces. He is not a rebel but a manipulative re-enactor of social gender stereotypes. The island is "hardly an island at low tide" and the malign system that Frank's father places on him relates to that of the mainland. Frank's "factory," his "Bomb Circle" and his hatred of women and nature are echoes of the larger society that his father supposedly rejects. Frank's discovery at the end of the book that he is "a normal female" reveals the extent to which "he" has internalized a cultural disgust at female anatomy: "Part of me still wants to believe it's just his latest lie, but really I know it's the truth. I'm a woman. Scarred thighs, outer labia a bit chewed up, and I'll never be attractive, but according to Dad a normal female, capable of intercourse and giving birth (I shiver at the thought of either)." In this imagined case, social gender reassignment has encouraged body dysphoria, specifically hatred of the female body. The rebel recreates the oppressive institutions and beliefs that he claims to reject. In this sense, Banks anticipates the ways in which transgender ideology echoes and reinforces social gender stereotypes.

When Prophecy Fails

In a now famous 1956 study *When Prophecy Fails*, Leon Festinger explored the techniques by which believers reconstruct their world in the aftermath of a promised apocalypse, a process he believed to be emblematic of any dramatic threat to our belief system: "The faithful could just as easily be those who stubbornly stand by disgraced politicians, failed ideologies, dishonest friends, or cheating spouses, even when reality highlights the clearest of inconsistencies" (Festinger et al, 2012). The revelation of Frank's true sex at the end of *The Wasp Factory* forces the reader to think back through the narrative and revise the story in retrospect. We thought we were reading the story of a boy; we revisit and rewrite the narrative as a story about a girl. It is hard to understand that the violence that is described is the work of a girl raised as a boy, for this story counters our beliefs about gender. As reader, no longer author of David Reimer's gender story, John Money faced a revision which threatened his professional authority. Money's get out clause was his insistence that the Reimer parents must never tell Brenda the truth for, just as in *The Wasp Factory*, treatment depended on a lie. Whilst some colleagues disowned Money after it was revealed that he had continue to publish the experiment as a success, some continued to defend him, including his collaborator Richard Green (2004) who explained that:

> "With the benefit of hindsight, based on what we knew at the time about how you become male or female or boy or girl, with the advantage of hindsight knowing the difficulties to say the least of creating a penis surgically, the decision that John Money made at the time was the correct one. And I would have made the same one at the time."

The phrase Green uses three times ("at the time") marks the shifting ground on which gender science rests. Although Money claimed that his theory had always allowed a role for prenatal hormonal exposure, the Reimer case helped to establish a new theory of gender identity as a deeply felt internal sense of self. Reimer somehow knew he was male, despite the way he was raised. What didn't change, though, was the therapeutic protocol that Money had established and made his own. Whereas Money claimed that gender identity was the central truth on which psychological coherence rested, in his own case, professional identity was revealed to be equally crucial to psychic survival. We might say that he was of the "psychiatrist gender."

For Judith Butler, the academic philosopher and gender theorist whose work is central to queer theory, the Reimer story offered a different kind of challenge. Butler (1990: 188) saw gender as the production of language and culture and rejected "both the expressive model of gender and the notion of a true gender identity." She does not use the concept of the "authentic self" which is now central to the language of transactivism but sees the "figure of the interior soul understood as 'within' the body" as the effect of power which creates "the illusion of an interior and organizing gender core" (Butler 1990: 184-186). Butler (2004) therefore rejects Colapinto's assumption that the Reimer story proves that nature trumps nurture. Instead, she effectively recruits Reimer's experience for a transsexual (not a transgender) narrative, pointing out that his reconstructed "neophallus" is a product of the medical technologies invented for transsexual patients. Butler differs from today's transactivists both insofar as she focuses on the body - on the surgery that Reimer both suffered and chose – but also insofar as she rejects the notion of an inner gender identity. For Butler, Reimer's experience turns into a fable of gender fluidity achieved through two transitions:

> we might say that Brenda/David together went through two transsexual surgeries: the first based on a hypothetical argument about what gender should be, given the ablated nature of the penis; the second based on what the gender should be, based on the behavioural and verbal indications of the person in question.

She finds something inspiring in his refusal to be defined by his genitals, seeing him as developing "a lay critique of the phallus". In a utopian conclusion, she describes David Reimer as an image of a future which escapes gender identities: "he is the human in its anonymity, as that which we do not yet know how to name or that which sets a limit on all naming." For Butler, Reimer expands the definition of what it is to be human, rejecting both Colapinto's and Money's assumption that gender identity is key.

But trans utopias are easier to write than to live and Butler's essay appears with a Postscript: "As this book was going to press in June of 2004, I was saddened to learn that David Reimer took his life at the age of 38." At this moment, Butler's theory – like Money's – confronts the resistance of a narrative twist it did not expect or intend. Like the ending of *The Wasp Factory*, this postscript sends the reader back to revisit what has been read, to ask how much has been taken for granted, how much simply misunderstood. In the light of this postscript, Butler's essay strikes a false note, taking Reimer – against his will – as a totemic example of her own gender utopia. Reimer, we now see, has been co-opted by Butler as part of her attempt at "Undoing Gender", the title of the collection which contains this essay.

Whose voice?

Frank, in *The Wasp Factory*, is an unreliable narrator who holds back his/her knowledge of her true sex, forcing the reader to live through the lie that her father imposed on her. Butler's (2004) most significant assumption is that Reimer (as recorded and transmitted by Colapinto) is also an unreliable narrator - even when describing his own experience. She points out that Reimer's understanding of gender manifests the influence of the conservative culture within which he was raised. And in this assumption, Butler is clearly correct. We know from Money's own account that Reimer was subject to strict gender policing:

> The effects of emphasizing feminine clothing became clearly noticeable in the girl's attitude towards clothes and hairdo [...] when she was observed to have a clear preference for dresses over slacks and to take a pride in her long hair. [...] Elsewhere in this same recorded interview, the mother said: "One thing that really amazes me is that she is so feminine. I've never seen a little girl so neat and tidy as she can be when she wants to be...She is very proud of herself, when she puts on a new dress, or I set her hair (Money and Ehrhardt 1996).

Butler quotes Reimer's account of his awakening to the truth of his gender: "I looked at myself and said I don't like this type of clothing, I don't like the types of toys I was always being given." But for her this moment of revelation does not provide narrative closure. Innocent of the possibility that stereotypes might be taken to reveal gender identity, Butler asks "in what world, precisely, do such dislikes count as clear or unequivocal evidence for or against being a given gender? Do parents regularly rush off to gender identity clinics when their boys play with yarn, or their girls play with trucks?" Our world, we might now answer.

Butler does not think that Reimer can know the truth of his own gender identity. She respects his account as "a self-description, and that is to be honoured. These are the words by which this individual gives himself to be understood." But she believes the self can only speak within the terms of a pre-existing discourse: "when one speaks, one speaks a language that is already speaking". The power that controls Reimer, in Butler's view, is that of a linguistic system that constrains meaning within categories formed by systems of power: David cannot stand up against the Goliath of discourse. Butler does not believe that adults can discover the gender identity of a child by listening to them, or by watching their behaviour.

Yet the injunction to "Listen to the kids" is central to the transgender ideology that has rapidly become hegemonic over the last five years. Here is the BBC's summary of a 2016 interview with a "non-binary" 10-year-old:

> Leo is 10 years old. For most of his life he's lived as a girl, but this summer he began to speak openly about his sense that this didn't feel quite right. With research help for his parents, he's decided he is non-binary - in his case, both masculine and feminine - though for the moment he dresses as a boy and has taken a male name. This is Leo's story in his own words (BBC 2016).

Phrases like "speak openly" and "in his own words" demand that we believe a 10-year-old to be capable of conceptualizing and communicating a gendered identity which escapes the limiting terms of his society. But this may be, as Butler says, Leo speaking "a language that is already speaking", a language in this case provided by his parents.

In *The Wasp Factory* Frank's unreliable narration speaks from within his father's misogynist gender ideology: "Both sexes can do one thing specially well", Frank, the narrator tells us: "women can give birth and men can kill. We – I consider myself an honorary man – are the harder sex. [...] I can feel it in my bones, in my uncastrated genes'. Although he considers himself a rebel, Frank's father is a product of the wider culture he inhabits, a culture that also forms Frank's view of gender:

> Women, I know from watching hundreds – maybe thousands – of films and television programmes, cannot withstand really major things happening to them; they get raped, or their loved ones die, and they go to pieces, go crazy and commit suicide, or just pine away until they die.

In Banks's novel, children do not speak their own words but ventriloquize the culture that produces them. Whereas transactivists insist on listening to the "voice of the child," Banks – like Butler - insists that children exist within the force field of a culture formed by adults. It is for this reason that they are uniquely in need of protection lest they be co-opted as unwitting actors in adult narratives.

Fiction, truth and lies

The Intersex Society of North America (ISNA) campaigns against "unwanted genital surgeries for people born with an anatomy that someone decided is not standard for male or female" and their website offers a simple and cogent reading of the Reimer case: that lies hurt. Money thanked "hermaphrodites or intersexes" for enabling his insight into "this new meaning of gender" and wrote that "To them social science and social history overall owe a debt of gratitude." (Money and Ehrhardt, 1996: xii). But at just this time intersex activists who felt that they had been harmed by Money's ideas were establishing a new set of ground rules: "For newborns with confusing sexual anatomy, assign a best-guess preliminary gender label of boy or girl, with the understanding that no surgery is required for a gender label." Because Money's treatment of Reimer followed his protocol for intersex babies, Reimer's story has become important to the intersex movement: "We like to point out that what the story of David Reimer teaches us most clearly is how much people are harmed by being lied to and treated in inhumane ways." (Intersex Society of North America, undated). Their key demand is "Above all, tell people the truth."

This reading of the Reimer case depends on sorting truth from lies. By contrast, the post-modern assumption that knowledge is made from multiple competing stories that are equally valid removes the opposition between truth and lie. Although Butler (2004) rejects the concept of a true gender identity, she cannot see that Reimer was hurt by Money's lies. Her theme is "the power of regulation, a power that determines, more or less, what we are, what we can be". But she will not adjudicate or stand in judgement:

> So what does my analysis imply? Does it tell us whether the gender here is true or false? No. And does this have implications for whether David should have been surgically transformed into Brenda or Brenda surgically transformed into David? No, it does not (Butler 2004:70).

Butler's post-modern relativism is now central to medical practice. The NHS Gender Identity Service at the Tavistock clinic which works with young people avoids "trying to work out who is 'right' or 'wrong'" (GIDS, 2017). Historian Alice Dreger is unusual in her insistence not only that evidence matters but also that there is such a thing as a right or wrong answer. It is not surprising, then, that Dreger's research focused on the definition of hermaphroditism in the nineteenth century and led to campaigning work with intersex activists. She argues passionately against academic relativism:

> What privilege such people enjoy who can say there is no objective reality, no way to ascertain more accurate knowledge! I know from experience, these are people who typically claim to speak on behalf of the marginalized and the oppressed, yet they have not sat and learned enough anatomy and medicine to know what a clitoroplasty actually involves in terms of loss of tissue and sensation; they have not witnessed what happens to the minds and bodies of scholars falsely accused of crimes against humanity (Dreger 2016:259).

A similar call for truth has been made by a small group of trans women who reject the activist claim that "trans women are women" because it "primes trans women for failure, disappointment, and cognitive dissonance." For these "gender apostates" the claim is "a lie that sets us up to be triggered every time we are called he, or 'guys' or somebody dares to suggest that we have male biology" (Goldberg, 2015). "Post-truth" was the Oxford Dictionaries' "word of the year 2016," an adjective "denoting circumstances in which objective facts are less influential in shaping public opinion than appeals to emotion and personal belief." Contemporary transgender doctrine relies centrally on an appeal to personal belief coupled with an emotional appeal to protect the oppressed. It is the product of a "post-truth" world.

    This chapter has argued that contemporary transgender ideology is a product of our moment in history, that it invents a new set of beliefs that are without historical precedent. It suggests that our new understanding of gender relies on semantic changes that can be traced over the last two hundred years. These changes can be seen in the stories produced by novelists, historians, gender theorists, psychiatrists and scientists. But it also asserts that stories are not all equally true. Plato (1993:71) may have been right to claim that there are "two kinds of literature, true and false" and that a society needs to distinguish between them in its education of the young: "Shall we, then, casually allow our children to listen to any old stories, made up by just anyone, and to take into their minds views which, on the whole, contradict those we'll want them to have as adults?" Stories can allow us to glimpse the narrowly circumscribed assumptions within which our culture represents the complexities of human experience: Gore Vidal's *Myra Breckinbridge* (a story of sex change) is one of the "rare gifts" presented to Frank by his father in *The Wasp Factory*, a book that Frank "assiduously avoided reading" though it might have allowed him to see through his father's lies.

But stories do not necessarily tell the truth, whether they are the work of novelists or sexologists, gender theorists or the BBC. One of the now forgotten categories of historical madness was "madness through literary identification," the common eighteenth century belief that susceptible readers could become mad when they failed to distinguish the world of fiction from that of reality. Fiction itself warns against this danger in *Don Quixote* or Charlotte Lennox's *The Female Quixote* or Austen's *Northanger Abbey*. The sane reader was one who could distinguish between the freedom of the imagination and the constraints of the real. And this warning is as pertinent to the 1818 *Frankenstein* which imagined technologies for overcoming the impassable barrier of death as to the twentieth century novel's fantasies of sex change and gender reversal. In the twenty-first century, gender has often taken over from religion to offer liberation from manifold forms of distress. But like earlier religious narratives, gender stories can lead to despair. At the end of the eighteenth century, the poet William Cowper's despair was triggered by a dream in which he heard a voice announcing his damnation (Cecil, 1929). In 2013, the blogger Zinnia Jones explains dysphoria in terms of gender: "Some of us suffer the distress that stems from dysphoria, but without many clues that this is about gender, and its relation to our genders may be obvious only in retrospect" (Jones 2013). Dysphoria (literally just unhappiness) is presumed to be driven by gender. Banks's story ends with the discovery of a "golden path" to a new freedom:

> Each of us, in our own personal Factory, may believe we have stumbled down one corridor, and that our fate is sealed and certain (dream or nightmare, humdrum or bizarre, good or bad), but a word, or glance, a slip – anything can change that, alter it entirely, and our marble hall becomes a gutter, or our rat-maze a golden path.

Escape from the body factory depends on recognising the fictional status of gender ideology.

References

Angier, N. (1997) *Sexual Identity Not Pliable After All, Report Says,* New York Times, March 14th
http://www.nytimes.com/1997/03/14/us/sexual-identity-not-pliable-after-all-report-says.html

Banks, I. (1984) *The Wasp Factory*, London: Abacus

BBC Magazine (2016) *I'm a non-binary 10-year-old,* 18th September 2016
http://www.bbc.co.uk/news/magazine-37383914

Bristow, J. (2010) *Sexuality*, London: Routledge
Butler, J. (1990) *Gender Trouble: Feminism and the Subversion of Identity*, New York and London: Routledge
—. (2004) *Undoing Gender*, New York and London: Routledge
Cameron, D. (2016) *Language: A Feminist Guide*. https://debuk.wordpress.com/2016/12/15/a-brief-history-of-gender
Cecil, D. (1929) *The Stricken Deer or The Life of Cowper*, London: Constable
Colapinto, J. (2013) *As Nature Made Him: The Boy that was Raised a Girl*, New York and London: Harper Perennial
Dreger, A. (2015) *Galileo's Middle Finger: Heretics, Activists, and one Scholar's Search for Justice*, New York: Penguin
Du Preez, M. and Dronfield, J. (2016) *Dr James Barry: A Woman Ahead of Her Time*, London: One World
Festinger, L., Riecken, H. and Schachter, S. (2012) *When Prophecy Fails*, Minneapolis: University of Minnesota Press
Foucault, M. (1978) *The History of Sexuality: The Will to Knowledge, London*: Penguin
GIDS (2017) *Gender Identity Development Service*, http://gids.nhs.uk/parents
Goldberg, M. (2015) *The Trans Women Who Say That Trans Women Aren't Women* http://www.slate.com/articles/double_x/doublex/2015/12/gender_critical_trans_women_the_apostates_of_the_trans_rights_movement.html
Goldie, T. (2014) *The Man Who Invented Gender: Engaging the Ideas of John Money*, Vancouver: University of British Columbia Press
Green, R. (2014) *Dr Money and the Boy with No Penis*, http://www.bbc.co.uk/sn/tvradio/programmes/horizon/dr_money_trans.shtml
Hayward, C. (2015) *"No One Was 'Gay' In The 18th Century: Why We Must Not Rewrite History with Today's Terms"*, New Statesman, 2nd March 2015, http://www.newstatesman.com/culture/2015/03/no-one-was-gay-18th-century-why-we-must-not-rewrite-history-today-s-terms.
Hobson, C. Z. (2000) *Blake and Homosexuality*, New York and Basingstoke: Palgrave
Intersex Society of North America (undated) *Who was David Reimer (also, sadly, known as 'John/Joan')?* http://www.isna.org/faq/reimer
Jackson, H.J. (2015) *Coleridge's Way With Words*, http://blog.oup.com/2015/08/samuel-coleridge-language

Jones, Z. (2013) *'That Was Dysphoria?' 8 Signs and Symptoms of Indirect Gender Dysphoria*, http://the-orbit.net/zinniajones/2013/09/that-was-dysphoria-8-signs-and-symptoms-of-indirect-gender-dysphoria/

Millett, K. (2000) *Sexual Politics*, Urbana and Chicago: University of Illinois Press

Money, J. and Ehrhardt, A. (1996) *Man & Woman, Boy & Girl: Gender Identity from Conception to Maturity*, Northvale N.J.: Jason Aronson Inc

Norton, R. (1992) *Mother Clap's Molly House: The Gay Subculture in England, 1700-1830*, London: Gay Men's Press

Plato (1993) *Republic*, Oxford: Oxford University Press

Preves, S. E. (2002) "Sexing the Intersexed: An Analysis of Sociocultural Responses to Intersexuality." *Signs,* 27 (2), 523-556

Pulver, A. (2016) *Rachel Weisz To Play Real-Life Gender-Fluid Victorian Doctor,* Guardian, 13 December 2016, https://www.theguardian.com/film/2016/dec/13/rachel-weisz-stars-james-barry-film-gender-fluid-victorian-doctor

Reid, R.W. (1994) *Orchidectomy As a Preliminary Procedure Prior to Gender Reassignment Surgery,* GENDYS conference, http://www.gender.org.uk/conf/1994/reid94.htm

Smith, B. R. (2000) "Premodern Sexualities," *PMLA*, Volume 115: 3 pp.318-329

Stryker, S. (2008) *Transgender History*, Berkeley: Seal Press

Watkins, E. S. (2007) *The Estrogen Elixir: A History of Hormone Replacement Therapy in America,* Baltimore: Johns Hopkins University Press

CHAPTER EIGHT

A FULL LIFE UNINTERRUPTED BY TRANSITION

MIRANDA YARDLEY

A Note on Language

Language within this field, like any political arena, can be fraught with difficulty and sensitivity, not least because language is sometimes used to obscure meaning. In the interests of clarity and consistency, the use of the word "transgender" is always used as an umbrella term to describe anyone of a range of identities whereby someone claims to "identify" with a sex class other than which they were born into. The word "transsexual" is more tightly defined, being someone who undertakes a surgical, medical and social transition in order to attempt to live permanently as a member of the sex opposite to which they are born. Natal or biological sex is always inferred from female or male, so a "transgender female" would be a natal female who claimed a "male identity" and "transgender male" a natal male who claimed a "female identity". Likewise, a "transsexual female" would be a natal female who has transitioned to live "as a man" and "transsexual male" a natal male who has transitioned to live "as a woman".

A Modern Epidemic

In the UK, the national centre for the assessment and treatment of gender dysphoric children and young adults is the Tavistock and Portman NHS Foundation Trust. In 2009/10, the number of referrals of males was 56 with 40 referrals of females, with a single referral of a child "of transsexual parent" with no apparent attempt to identify sex, total 97, split 58.3% male and 41.7% female. (The Tavistock and Portman NHS Foundation Trust, 2016).

In 2011/12 the number of females referred surpassed males and this remained so for each subsequent year until the latest reported figures for 2015/16 which show a total of 1,419 referrals split between 490 male and 929 female and a shift in composition to 65.5% female and 34.5% male. This represents a huge increase in the numbers of children and young adults seeking help for gender non-conformity and cross-sex identification, as well as a significant change in the sex composition of children and young adults seeking help; historically, the reported incidences of males seeking such help has far outstripped the numbers of females, yet this appears to no longer be the case.

Is it unreasonable to ask why it is that there has been a fifteen-fold increase in referrals of children and young people over a six year period, and why does this represent a 23-fold increase in girls against just an 8.75 increase in boys? Why in 2015/16 have referrals of children aged eight or younger risen to 101, compared to ten in 2009/10, with twenty aged five or less (2009/10 – six), with no apparent reason offered to explain these changes?

If this were as result of a pathogen, there's little doubt it would be treated as an epidemic. Within this chapter, the argument will be made that the vector motivating these increases originates from a group whose interests and histories are unrelated to these children. It will also be shown that both the existing scientific knowledge we have about the etiology of transsexualism and further enquiry and debate around this are being prevented by that same group through tactics of threats and intimidation.

What is the etiology of "transgender identity"?

The Tavistock and Portman "Gender Identity Development Service" (GIDS) runs a specialist website under its own marque. The remit of the GIDS is explained as follows:

> We recognise how complex ideas around gender can be and that there is a huge range of human diversity in how people feel about and express their gender. Young people who are developing an understanding of their own gender that is different from what everyone had first expected can sometimes find things very tough. Both young people and their families can experience high levels of distress as their gender identity evolves.
> (The Tavistock and Portman NHS Foundation Trust, 2016)

On the GIDS website, the service freely admits it is at a loss as to why any children would be struggling with their 'gender' or 'gender identity' indeed the website's own glossary makes no attempt to define either:

> If you are asking about why you are questioning your gender or why you feel that you are transgender, then the honest answer is we do not know exactly why this happens to some people... some people feel strongly that they are "born this way" when it come to their gender identity, and they might find the idea of having, for example, "a boy's brain in a girl's body" helpful in explaining their experience... we know that how people experience and show their gender, and how people respond to gender non-conformity, is linked to the culture and the time in which they live.
> (The Tavistock and Portman NHS Foundation Trust, 2016)

A section on 'current debates' hints:

> Young people are understanding gender in an increasingly diverse way. For example, Facebook now allows users to choose from an "extensive list" of pre-populated gender identities, or to enter their own preferred terms. Each individual can add up to 10 terms describing their gender to their profile and can customise how public this information is made. Young people who we meet at GIDS have often familiarised themselves with a large range of different identity labels in discussions online or with their peers.
> (The Tavistock and Portman NHS Foundation Trust, 2016)

The existence of cultural aspects of gender is acknowledged, for example the cultural response to non-conformity and the effect of a shifting understanding of what 'gender' means to young people. Yet these pages leave the reader with little apparent understanding of why it is that anyone would be transgender. Is this really the case? Are transgender individuals "born this way"? Is it meaningful to talk of "a boy's brain in a girl's body"?

What is gender?

In common use, the word "gender" is often taken to be associated with sex, we talk of gendered clothing, toys or even nouns, and these are coded as masculine, feminine or even neutral. Of course, we don't mean that the clothing, toys or nouns are actually male or female, what we mean is that these are culturally associated with the state of being male or female; these cultural ideas are attached to a particular sex by culture. And this is what is meant when feminists say that gender is socially, or culturally, constructed, that it is a result of society imposing what is culturally acceptable upon a particular sex. A distinction may therefore be drawn between sex, as a biological state, and gender as cultural norms associated with that state. The World Health Organisation separates sex and gender as follows:

> "Sex" refers to the biological and physiological characteristics that define men and women. "Gender" refers to the socially constructed roles, behaviours, activities, and attributes that a given society considers appropriate for men and women. To put it another way: "Male" and "female" are sex categories, while "masculine" and "feminine" are gender categories. Aspects of sex will not vary substantially between different human societies, while aspects of gender may vary greatly.
> (World Health Organisation, undated)

Sex distinctions exist outside of culture, but what exists within the convention of gender exists only because human beings say so; this is why we say that gender is socially constructed. Biological sex itself is a material reality, membership of a sex class is based upon perceived reproductive potential as producers of large gametes (female, child-bearers) or small gametes (males, those who impregnate the child-bearers). The biological consequences of being a member of each sex follow.

A small number of individuals are born with an intersex condition. These are a result of chromosomal or genetic abnormalities. A body is taken to be 'chromosomally male' if it the body's cells have a Y chromosome, however the masculinisation of features may not happen because of, for example, SRY abnormalities (on the gene itself) or through androgen insensitivity syndrome (where the body does not respond to expressed androgens). In this case, male bodies are apparent with female primary sex characteristics and the underlying sex of the individual generally only comes to be recognised after investigation, usually in the teenage years. There are other chromosomal abnormalities affecting males for example XYY, XXY, XXXY and even XXXXY, it should be noted these are still male by the Y chromosome, and many such males successfully father children.

The examples of gender quoted by the WHO illustrate a factor about gender leading to the "feminist analysis of gender". Of the four examples chosen, three have negative consequences for women (although an example about smoking is negative, in that "smoking has not traditionally been considered appropriate" shows that in Viet Nam the prohibition on women smoking may be culturally interpreted as being negative). The feminist interpretation of gender is that it is a hierarchical system used to oppress women, as the positive and active stereotypes are reserved for the men while negative and submissive stereotypes are imposed upon women.

When transgender individuals talk about gender, it is usually in the context of "gender identity". This term arose in psychoanalysis (Stoller, 1964) which defines "gender identity" as follows:

> Gender identity is the sense of knowing to which sex one belongs, that is, the awareness "I am a male" or "I am a female"… (g)ender identity seems to be produced in normal human beings by the following elements: first, the anatomy and physiology of the external genital organs, by which is meant the appearance of and the sensations from the external, visible, and palpable genitalia; second, the attitudinal influences of parents, siblings, and peers. Whether these consider a child a boy or a girl will ordinarily play an extremely important part in establishing and confirming the gender identity.

Stoller's definition is primarily based upon the biology of the subject, and secondly upon cultural aspects, and underlining the importance of the influence of "parents, siblings and peers". A typical definition from a transgender support group would be as follows:

> One's innermost concept of self as male or female or both or neither - how individuals perceive themselves and what they call themselves. One's gender identity can be the same or different than the sex assigned at birth. Individuals are conscious of this between the ages 18 months and 3 years. Most people develop a gender identity that matches their biological sex. For some, however, their gender identity is different from their biological or assigned sex.
> (Gender Spectrum, 2016)

This separates the concept of "gender identity" from biological reality and the child's social environment, which as Stoller defined it is foundational upon the perception of that child's sex by "parents, siblings and peers", and appears to suggest this identity is something else, which one becomes aware of as consciousness matures. It states that the developed "gender identity" may be different from the child's sex but is silent to the mechanism, implying this may be a matter of luck (or misfortune).

When transgender individuals speak of their "gender" it is usually taken to mean the internal sense of self, rather than the external reality of what that person physically may be. A consequence of this is that it is not uncommon to encounter masculine males, sometimes fathers, claiming to be female based upon how they feel inside, yet everything else about them suggests otherwise, they may have a flowing beard. This is, of course, an extreme; there are many individuals who are female (or male) who identify as members of the opposite sex and, it could be argued, bear more of a resemblance to those whom they claim to identify with. This 'gender expression' is often through behaviour, clothes and personal grooming, and with transsexuals accompanied with the external intervention of synthetic hormones or even surgery upon the genitals, torso, face and hairline. Is this, though, what makes 'a woman', or 'a man'?

In her 1949 book 'The Second Sex', the French philosopher Simone de Beauvoir famously wrote:

> One is not born, but rather becomes, a woman. (de Beauvoir, 1949)

de Beauvoir with Jean-Paul Sartre founded the existentialist philosophical movement. Existentialism does not presuppose that we have an innate soul or essence; rather what we are is the sum of our opportunities and experiences. There is no 'female essence' or 'male essence' or spirit, and a philosophically honest interpretation of de Beauvoir's words are that being a woman is a whole life experience based upon her biology, the effect of being a woman in a world of men, and what society does to her.

Although a woman may be taken as 'an adult human female', words often have more than one meaning and this reflects what de Beauvoir was getting at; she becomes what she is through being a woman living in a world within the system of gender. Making a distinction between sex and gender, it makes a woman a product of both her sex and of the system of gender (Butler, 1986).

It is interesting to examine the commonalities between the lives and experiences of those who claim a "transgender" identity. Historically, stories that made the media consisted mainly of adult males who announced to the world their new identity, however recently we are seeing more evidence of young children and adolescents as well as females "transitioning" to male. We will look first at the narratives of transgender children ("transkids") and then transgender adults ("adult transitioners").

Commonality in the "transkids" narrative

The narratives of children that are claimed to be transgender are startlingly similar. Based upon a review of a small sample of 'human interest' stories on the Daily Mail website (a widely-read conservative British newspaper) which told the stories of these children and their parents, the histories of young transgender males (boys who 'want' to be girls) show a strong consistency on a number of points which may be taken as culturally stereotyped behaviour of boys and girls. For example, these included a preference for pink (7/7 cases), feminine hair (6/7), playing princesses and wearing dresses (5/7), preferences for 'toys for girls' (5/7) (Yardley, 2017).

This narrative is not unique to the source. Interviewed in 2015, Susie Green, CEO of the transgender children's charity Mermaids Gender recounted a similar narrative for her son Jack, who has transitioned to Jackie (Albert, 2015) and is reflected in another significant narrative on the British National Health Service website (NHS Choices, 2009). In the latter case, the parent procured testosterone blockers for her son from a doctor in the USA when the child was just thirteen.

A review of equivalent narratives for transgender girls (natal females) suggests a different emphasis. In contrast to the transgender boys, who usually are pre-teens, the age of the subject is often old enough for them to be able to indicate their sexual orientation which shows itself to be the striking commonality; in each of the four narratives reviewed, prior to transition the girl has identified as a homosexual female, a lesbian (Yardley, 2017).

Although other cultural preferences are evident for boys, every single one of those narratives indicates a childhood preference for pink. The nature of pink for girls and blue for boys is cultural and so changes, both across cultures and through time, indeed gender-neutral clothing was popular until around 1985 when gender-specific clothing became identified as being another way businesses could make money out of parents, "the more you individualize clothing, the more you can sell" with the availability of prenatal testing being a major motivator (Maglaty, 2011).

Devoid of culture, pink has no meaning with respect to the preferences of children, or even adults, of either sex. Notably in the stories for young transgender females, many include a rejection of pink, dresses and princesses, the diametric opposite of the stories from transgender males. As noted above the transgender females shared homosexual sexual orientation. This has been noted by feminist commentators who have framed the transitioning of young girls and boys as a form of gay eugenics:

> There are many lesbians today who say that if gender identity politics were as prevalent when they were young as they are now, that instead of growing up to recognise and embrace their gender non-conformity and same-sex attraction, they would have thought they were boys... (i)ndeed, there are many critics of transactivism who say that this new trend for medicating young people on the basis of gender identity is a form of gay eugenics... Transactivist Scout Barbour-Evans said, himself, on Radio

Live, that gender is a "social construct", and he was right about that. And when young people are medicated, to the point of sterilisation, just to better align with and conform to social constructs – that is eugenics. And because gender conformity has so much to do with compulsory heterosexuality – it's a form of gay eugenics.
(Gerlich, 2017)

If we can accept that "gender identity" is a preference for the cultural conventions applicable to a particular sex, is it such a leap to suggest that for girls who are masculine (or boys who are feminine), such personality traits are being interpreted as an indicator that the child's "gender identity" is not correspondent with the child's sex? Is this not tantamount to suggesting that personality determines sex? Of course, children's preferences can change suddenly and just as cultural ideas of gender are not stable over time, neither is the gender non-conforming behaviour of children. In a review of eleven follow-up studies from 1972 to 2013, James Cantor concluded that 60–90% of trans- kids turn out no longer to be trans by adulthood (Cantor, 2016).

If we can agree that masculinity in females is socially coded as being lesbian and femininity in males is socially coded as gay (as Gerlich observes) there is a real danger that gender non-confirming behaviour in children is being interpreted not as this being a child who will grow up to be homosexual, rather our feminine boys and masculine girls are being perceived to be and treated as being "transgender". Should children continue to transition at the increasing rates we have been seeing, there is a danger this will annihilate our lesbian and gay population.

Do later transitioners follow the 'transkids' narrative?

We can compare the narratives of transsexuals who did not transition young and establish what if any commonality there is between each of these, and the narratives claimed for the 'transkids'. Taking the frank, published accounts of three male transsexuals who did not transition as children, none of whom identify as 'homosexual transsexuals' (whose romantic/sexual history is stated as either bisexual or heterosexual), we can see there is another force with some types of transsexual that differs from those claimed by 'transkids'.

In 'Other Lands' (Roche, 2016) a powerful piece from someone who transitioned in their forties, the author details their experiences shortly after gender reassignment surgery (creation of a neo-vagina through a surgical process on penile tissue). In place of the descriptions of stereotypically feminine behaviours and preferences from young children, we have the recollection of teenage fantasy, describing the author's erotic dream of having female genitals, and the description of their own or other person's interaction with this feminised version of the young man they were. The language used is overly sexual, seemingly colloquial to pornography, with the vagina described as a "moist slit" and the plea, 'Silence of the Lambs'-style, "I'm a beautiful pussy fuck me."

Another piece talks of the consumption of transgender pornography (Williams, 2016) which had followed a history of cross-dressing fetishism:

> I did have a history of cross-dressing fetishism, with a particular predilection for nylon. In a nutshell, I would wear women's clothing and become aroused... In high school and college, I discovered porn with trans women. If I was having sexual fantasies at all back then, it was probably about trans women, not myself as a woman with a vagina living in a female gender role... I eventually came to realize that the reason I was so fascinated by trans woman porn was that I was projecting myself into the bodies of the trans women as I watched and identifying with them. I realized over time that I wanted the body of a non-op trans woman. I liked that aesthetic. I wanted that for myself. I am becoming what I love.

Another piece discusses how the author discovered their transgender identity:

> Anyone who knew me growing up knew that I was fascinated with women. I was the first of my friends to think that Playboy was a must-have magazine; I even remember begging my mom to buy me a copy for my 10th birthday... my interest wasn't just erotic. What I was never able to explain until recently was the confusion in my head between being attracted to a beautiful woman, and wanting to actually be one. As a result, I spent so many years wondering if I was the only guy that felt this way, or if all guys did and no one was willing to talk about it. But it turns out, that like sexual preference, gender identity is also a spectrum. (Egan, 2016)

The internet is rife with narratives connecting the consumption of pornography, particularly involving transgender people and self-realisations of being transgender. For example, in a thread on Reddit "Question About Porn" the answers posted to the question "Did anybody masturbate to transgender porn before they realized they were trans?" drew an almost unanimously positive response (Reddit.com, 2016). There are strong erotic aspects within each of these narratives and fantasy-based visualisations of the transsexual male as having female anatomy. These narratives have little in common with the 'transkids' narrative, yet certainly do themselves share commonality: there is an influence of pornography either intimated through use of language, explicitly admitted and even hypothesised as motivation for transition.

The Two-Type Model of Transsexualism

The existence of an erotic component to a type of transsexualism has been documented for over a hundred years where what was described as an 'automonosexualism streak' amongst transvestites was identified that was not just confined to cross-dressing (Hirshfeld, 1918). Existence of two discrete types of transsexual, differentiated by sexual orientation and age was hypothesised sixty years later (Buhrich, 1978) and it was suggested that transsexualism more common in males than females because of fetishist arousal through cross-dressing. It was also suggested that even among fetishistic cross-dressers, there were discrete behavioural types.

In 1985, sexologist Ray Blanchard suggested that there exists a fundamental difference between homosexual transsexuals (homosexual males romantically and sexually attracted to males) and non-homosexual transsexuals (which includes heterosexual, bisexual and asexual transsexuals) and on this basis there are two different types of transsexual differentiated by sexual orientation: transsexuals may be grouped into homosexual and non-homosexual transsexuals, and that the latter group contains a number of subtypes which could be taken to correspond to an ordinal degree of fetishistic transvestisism. These observations are supported by empirical evidence; the difference is manifest in "a much higher proportion of fetishistic cases than the homosexual group" and so Blanchard confirms the identification of two types of male transsexual, who are differentiated by sexual orientation, with one group displaying a fetishistic, or paraphilic history (Blanchard, 1985).

Blanchard became a key figure in the history of investigation into transsexualism a few years later where he attempted to impart meaning and rigor into the terminology surrounding the taxonomy of transsexuals, as part of systematic study into this phenomenon, he coined the term "autogynephilia" as a clearer description of something that had hitherto been described as part of automonosexualism. This is what has become known as "Blanchard's transsexual typology" or the "two-type transsexual typography" (Blanchard, 1989).

Autogynephilia is not something that is always on the mind, nor is it something that is confined solely to cross-dressing. Furthermore, the fetishist cross-dresser can be, or become, gender dysphoric (Blanchard,

1989). Classifying this behaviour in terms that lie outside of transvestic fetishism allowed Blanchard to apply his systematic study to a wider spectrum of behaviour observed within transsexuals, and he explained the etymology of "autogynephilia" based upon "a male's propensity to be sexually aroused by the thought or image of himself as a female" (Blanchard, 1991) and identifies four different types of autogynephilic behaviour:

> Autogynephilic fantasies and behaviors may focus on the idea of exhibiting female physiologic functions, of engaging in stereotypically feminine behavior, of possessing female anatomic structures, or of dressing in women's apparel. The last-mentioned class of fantasies and behaviors represents the familiar form of autogynephilia, transvestism. All four types of autogynephilia tend to occur in combination with other types rather than alone. (Blanchard, 1991)

This typological framework allows researchers to model or systematically analyse the behaviours of male transsexuals that separates these into homosexual and non-homosexual transsexuals, the latter who tend to be autogynephilic and exhibits one or more types of paraphilic behaviours. Blanchard has compared these paraphilic behaviours to a sexual orientation (Blanchard, 1993).

The homosexual transsexuals are what one may consider the more 'classic' popular image of the transsexual, with the non-homosexual transsexuals making lives that encompass successful careers as men as well and marriages and children, before transitioning later in life (Lawrence, 2004); the homosexual transsexual and the non-homosexual transsexual have different lives and experiences, although there is commonality in they are both transsexual with similar levels of experienced gender dysphoria. Psychologist J Michael Bailey (Bailey, 2003) lamented:

> To anyone who has seen members of both types and who has learned to ask the right kinds of questions, it is easy to tell them apart. Yet the difference has eluded virtually everyone who cares about transsexuals: talk show hosts, journalists, most people who evaluate and treat them, and even most academics who have studied them... (t)he most interesting reason why most people do not realize that there are two types of transsexuals is that members of one type sometimes misrepresent themselves as members of the other. I will get more specific later, but for now, it is enough to say that they are often silent about their true motivation and instead tell stories about themselves that are misleading and, in important respects, false.

> From soon after birth, the homosexual male-to-female transsexual behaves and feels like a girl. Unlike most feminine boys... these transsexuals do not outgrow, or learn to hide, their femininity. Instead, they decide that the drastic step of changing their sex is preferable. They unambiguously desire and love men, especially heterosexual men, whom they can attract only as women... one type of transsexual man is a kind of homosexual man.
>
> Honest and open autogynephilic transsexuals reveal a much different pattern. They were not especially feminine boys. The first overt manifestation of what led to their transsexualism was typically during early adolescence, when they secretly dressed in their mothers' or sisters' lingerie, looked at themselves in the mirror, and masturbated. This activity continued into adulthood, and sexual fantasies became increasingly transsexual—especially the fantasy of having a vulva, perhaps being penetrated by a penis. Autogynephilic transsexuals might declare attraction to women or men, to both, or to neither. But their primary attraction is to the women that they would become.

Bailey's interpretation of the motivation to change sex of homosexual transsexuals is to attract heterosexual men; we could consider given the choice in a homophobic society of living as a feminine gay man or as a woman, the homosexual transsexual may opt for the latter. While identifying the autogynephile's motivation for many behaviours, he stops short of hypothesising why the autogynephile would transition; surely, the prospect of castration and removal of the penis would be an irrational course of action for someone whose sexual identity was so invested in this? This, however, would be based on the misconception that autogynephilia is exclusively erotic. Anne Lawrence suggested the autogynephile's motivation may be compared to romantic love (Lawrence, 2003):

> ... purely erotic aspects of autogynephilia have received the greatest emphasis, while the aspects related to "amatory propensity," "sexual orientation," and "love" have received comparatively little. Love has been conspicuously absent in most discussions of autogynephilia, whether by its advocates or by its critics... individuals are often especially inclined to seek out passionate love experiences, or to allow themselves the possibility of entering into them, in middle age and in times of crisis. This is consistent with the life histories of many, if not most, nonhomosexual MtF transsexuals, who tend to seek sex reassignment in their 40s or later, sometimes in association with a midlife crisis ... (t)heir decision to undergo sex reassignment is not uncommonly preceded by some significant loss or reversal, such as unemployment, physical disability, or the end of an important relationship... (f)or individuals who experience autogynephilia, deciding

to become what one loves can represent an attempt to cope with adverse life circumstances, just as deciding to pursue a love affair with another person can for individuals with more conventional sexual orientations… the process of changing one's body and living as a woman offers an identity, a program of action, and a purpose in life.

Interpretations of "gender identity" and autogynephilia

We have established a concept of "gender identity" being the individual's inner feeling of male or female, which is taken to be influenced by biology and cultural effects, for example how the individual is treated by the people around them (Stoller, 1964). Referring to a later paper (Stoller, 1968) Lawrence suggests claims that gender identity is set young in a biological and cultural context and that the "core gender identity" of non-homosexual is always male (Lawrence, 2013). A different interpretation is offered by Julia Serano in "Whipping Girl", Serano's "transfeminist manifesto" (Serano, 2007):

> When I hit puberty, my newly found attraction to women spilled into my dreams of becoming a girl. For me, sexuality became a strange combination of jealousy, self-loathing, and lust. Because when you isolate an impressionable transgender teen and bombard her with billboard ads baring bikini clad women and boys' locker room trash talk about this girl's tits and that girl's ass, then she will learn to turn her gender identity into a fetish… my thirteen-year-old brain started concocting scenarios straight out of SM handbooks. Most of my fantasies began with my abduction: I'd turn to putty in the hands of some twisted man who would turn me into a woman as part of his evil plan. It's called forced feminization, and it's not really about sex. It is about turning the humiliation you feel into pleasure, transforming the loss of male privilege into the best fuck ever.

Serano claims to visualise fantasies of having a female body as well as independently arsing forced feminisation fantasies. This is an interesting claim to make, in that Serano claims the embodiment fantasy may have been culturally motivated, turning their own "gender identity into a fetish" yet Serano also suggests their own feminisation fantasy to be not just *a priori*, but the resultant loss of male privilege is "the best fuck ever". In terms of the autogynephilia model, there is a co-existence of behavioural, transvestic fetishist and anatomical autogynephilia, and also note the use of language that is rather masculine. The apparent fetishisation of the loss of male privilege ("best fuck ever") is ideologically anti-feminist as it pictures the 'woman' as helpless and submissive, and based on Blanchard and Lawrence's observations unconvincing.

In spite of claiming such a narrative where they are literally discussing "becoming what they love", Serano takes the view that autogynephilia is itself stigmatising, and suggests a rebranding as "Female/Feminine Embodiment Fantasies (FEFs)" (Serano, 2015).

To counteract perceived stigmatisation of autogynephilia, it has been suggested the phenomena exists in women (Moser, 2009), this study makes a claims that in some cases 93% of women could be interpreted as being autogynephilic. The study is not without its critics: the survey questions which form the basis of the study are not directly comparable to those used to assess autogynephilia in males (Lawrence, 2017) and the data collection was based upon handing out fifty-one questionnaires in a hospital foyer at random, of which twenty-nine were returned, described as a "convenience sample". Owing to the non-random nature of this sample, inferences cannot be drawn (Price, 2013). At the heart of this work is a logical flaw; as autogynephilia is described in terms of a male bodied individual fantasising about a female body, behaviours, physiology or anatomy; attributing a (female bodied) woman fantasising about being female bodied does not appear to be comparing like for like (for example "I have dressed in lingerie, sexy attire or prepared myself shaving my legs, applying make-up, etc. before masturbating"). We may conclude that whatever this study is claiming, it is not "autogynephilia in women" (Dreger, 2015).

In support of his "two type model", Blanchard suggested there may be differences between the brain structures of male transsexuals and "typical heterosexual men", with homosexual transsexuals exhibiting sex-dimorphic structures, and differences with non-homosexual transsexuals that neither involve sex-dimorphic structures nor lie along the male-female dimension (Blanchard, 2008). Empirical investigation suggests this to be the case (Rametti, et al., 2010), (Savic & Arver, 2010), (Cantor, 2011) with transsexual brains being characterised based upon sexual orientation; transsexual homosexuals have a similar brain structure variation from transsexual heterosexuals in the same way that non-transsexual homosexuals vary from heterosexual transsexuals.

"Gender identity" as a concept is as we have seen not universally agreed and does itself have a number of philosophical problems, many of which arise from the use of the term in common language and through what are known as "identity politics" (Reilly-Cooper, 2015) although what Reilly-Cooper observes is more informed by inconsistencies in the way the term is used by those who claim such identities, and how these differ from how "gender identity" has been defined in the literature by reference to biological sex and socialisation (Stoller, 1964). Reilly-Cooper also comments on the essentialist and subjective nature of "innate gender identity", which is consistent with de Beauvoir's non-essentialist existential approach.

Reilly-Cooper draws a distinction between the two most common popular interpretations of what "being transgender" means, the idea of an unprovable "soul or some other non-material entity" and the idea of someone having the brain of one sex inhabiting the body of another. The argument about sexed brains and in particular the connection of cultural artefacts to innate biology merits a book of its own, much has been written on this matter, some of which include assessment of the methodology of the work that leads to such claims (Fine, 2010).

Blanchard has addressed what he called "the feminine essence theory" in some detail (Blanchard, 2008) setting out the "tenets" of such a theory based on his own observed observations of what has been claimed, in the absence of a single "official version". Summarising this "feminine essence theory", Blanchard makes some key observations, including what may be seen as a fundamental shift in what, for want of a better expression, may be described as "transgender ideology":

> The popular description of male-to-female transsexuals as women trapped in men's bodies has sometimes been interpreted to mean that they feel like women or that they wish to be women. The feminine essence theory proposes that they are women.

This echoes what has become the rallying cry of today's transgender rights movement, "trans women are women" which is justified as follows:

> the notion that there exist one or more sex-dimorphic structures of the human brain that can be regarded as the seat of gender identity, and that key parameters of these structures (e.g., neuron number or density) are similar in male-to-female transsexuals and natal females... Contemporary proponents of this view also generally hold that the female-typical structure of the gender identity center(s) is congenital, so that male-to-female transsexuals are and always have been female where it counts - in the brain.

This has commonality with another common claim, that of "sex is what is between the legs, gender is what is in the brain". With what Blanchard calls "singularity of the feminine essence", he demonstrates this idea is incompatible with a two-type model of transsexuals:

> Human females do not occur in alternative morphs... do not consist of two or more discrete subpopulations with different phenotypes... (s)ince there is only one type of human female, there can be only one type of female trapped in a male body. It follows that the notion of a taxonomy of transsexuals with discrete diagnostic categories is almost oxymoronic... (t)here is no more need to ask whether homosexual and heterosexual male-to-female transsexuals have the same reasons for believing themselves to be women than there is to ask whether homosexual and heterosexual natal females have the same reasons for believing themselves to be women.

As transsexual males who have spent most of their lives conforming to societal convention to act masculine thus demonstrate male traits, the existence of both male and female traits in transsexuals does not itself challenge the "feminine essence theory", however the theory *is* incompatible with a high incidence of distinctive traits that are neither male nor female coded. The high incidence of autogynephilia amongst male to female transsexuals does itself challenge the "feminine essence theory" indicates why transsexuals and their allies have sought to characterise autogynephilia as an expression of female sexuality (Moser, 2009) however Blanchard suggests the this is likely because of there being two distinctly different etiologies to each distinct type of transsexualism: (Blanchard, 2008).

Blanchard has considered the existence of a "third type" of transsexual and framed this within the context of body integrity identity disorder (BIID), noting the apparent absence of evidence to support this phenomena and connecting this to the common incidence of erotic arousal. He earlier noted the self-reported histories of both individuals with BIID and gender identity disorder distort their history (Blanchard, 2003). Ultimately, however, he considers the concept of a third type of transsexual unhelpful to this "feminine essence theory" as the corollary of this is there can only be one kind of "true transsexualism".

Although there have been attempts to discredit Blanchard's typology, these have individually and collectively failed to diminish the value of the two-type typology in separating the population of male transsexuals into two distinct groups based upon sexual orientation (Lawrence, 2017).

The flag-bearers of transgenderism

As we have already seen, the media loves a "transgender coming out story", and in particular it will run with sensational stories based on males who transition after making a career in a typically masculine profession. These stories are often high on affirmation and sensation, with little analysis as to what it means for a man who is in his sixties, and fathered children, to suddenly declare themselves to be 'a woman'. Contemporary examples of both these being boxing promoter Kellie (Frank) Maloney or reality television star and former athlete Caitlyn (Bruce) Jenner.

In 2014, boxing promoter Kellie Maloney was effectively forced by the British press to make their transition to Kellie public. Some of the press coverage echoed what has become the language of transgender advocacy. For example, writing in The Independent, transgender activist Paris Lees, under the headline "Kellie Maloney has always been female" suggested that Maloney had always been "a woman" because he "felt different inside" (Lees, 2014). There is no attempt made within the feature to justify these claims, despite the fact that Maloney was on their second marriage and had fathered three children inside these two marriages.

Early in 2015, former Olympic decathlete Bruce Jenner ended years of speculation by announcing they too would be undertaking a 'transition', although some months passed between the initial admission of their transition to be, a dramatic announcement came from the style magazine Vanity Fair which placed Jenner on the cover and, in a matter of a few hours, the newly opened Twitter account for Caitlyn Jenner amassed over a million followers. Lees followed this announcement with a gushing, uncritical feature in The Guardian under the headline "Caitlyn Jenner: a life-affirming, provocative and downright fabulous Vanity Fair cover" (Lees, 2015), even going so far as to paint Jenner a victim of a cruel society that would not allow that incredibly wealthy, successful man to live the life he wanted; in spite of having six children from three marriages, a career as a top-flight Olympic gold winning athlete winning gold at the 1976 Montreal Olympics in the decathlon, an event that was not (and still is) open to women, and a subsequent career in reality television we are expected to view the preceding sixty-five years of Jenner's life as being incomplete.

Writing in The Morning Star, my own take on this was different. The sexualised cover shot of Jenner is represents the end product of the industry that has grown to fulfil the demand for cosmetic surgery for transgender individuals, in this case someone whose consent to surgery was made after a life that by anyone else's standards would already have been both full and successful. Yet, we are now expected to believe that Jenner spent the last sixty-five years in torment, hiding the person they really are, and (for reasons unspecified) can only now become free. How do the lives of Jenner and Maloney relate to the lives of the fifty-two percent of the population born and raised as women? (Yardley, 2015).

In April 2014, Jenner was interviewed by Diane Sawyer on ABC news programme '20/20', and when questioned as to their motivations for transition, Jenner claimed ownership of a "female brain." The existence of inherently differently sexed male and female brains is scientifically contentious and there is no significant generally accepted evidence that points to neurological differences in males and females that would explain, for example, an affinity for pink (Maglaty, 2011) or wanting to wear a dress or makeup (Fine, 2010). Individual preferences for cultural artefacts do not exist in a vacuum and are meaningless without context. This display was summarised as follows (Yardley, 2015):

> Jenner is not a "gender outlaw" breaking down boundaries and a mechanism for positive change. Jenner represents the status quo, in opposition to the positive, progressive force and changes that decades of women's suffrage and activism have fought for... this image of Jenner as being not "a man becoming a woman" but... "a man becoming a man's idea of what a woman should be"... an idealised body is presented clothed only in lingerie, the makeup is done to perfection, and every flaw is magically Photo shopped out of existence. Pandering to the male gaze, the body language is coy, seductive, submissive. This is not liberation, this is not revolution, this is not life-affirming. This is the crass stereotyping of what it means to be a woman, meeting every reactionary, culturally conservative ideal of what a woman should be — passive, objectified, dehumanised.

We should not need to be reminded that Maloney and Jenner are very different types of transsexuals to our feminine, likely pre-homosexual boys. Yet these transitions are used within Lees's Guardian piece to argue in favour of children's transition with no indication given as to the etiology of someone "being transgender" or any acknowledgement there could be a reason for these adult's transition that is fundamentally different to what we are seeing with young children (Lees, 2015). The piece raises more questions than it answers: what sort of society makes people hide from the world who they are for most of their lives? How can a man who transitions in his 60s know anything about the lived life experience of "being a woman"? How can either have "always been a woman ... even when they were 'fathering' children"? How can these statements have any coherent meaning in what we know about ourselves, or the reproduction of other mammals? What do statements like this mean for homosexuals and homosexuality if, for example, a transgender male "identifies" as a lesbian? Is our understanding and acceptance of what it is to be homosexual now framed within a structure that now includes heterosexuals?

If the vectors that lead to the transition of children and adults are so different, why would anyone pretend different? The reason for this is, of course, because of what it means for the adults. Until publication of Bailey's book (Bailey, 2003) there was very little public knowledge of the existence of Blanchard's "two-type model" or the concept of "autogynepilia". There was an incredible backlash by a number of prominent American transgender activists that resulted in attempts to public discredit Bailey's work and unprecedented acts of harassment against him, his children and other members of his family. The events surrounding this were documented meticulously by Alice Dreger in "The Controversy Surrounding The Man Who Would Be Queen: A Case History of the Politics of Science, Identity, and Sex in the Internet Age" (Dreger, 2008), identifying the start of problems for Bailey first when his book was announced as a finalist for the Lambda Literary Award then cataloguing threats, intimidation, malicious communications to his employer and colleagues, and malicious content created on the internet alleging impropriety against his own children.

Lawrence contextualised attacks as a display of narcissistic rage (Lawrence, 2008), referencing earlier work by Kohut (Kohut, 1972) and characterising fanatic revenge as the response to narcissistic hurt. Lawrence makes a number of points which enable us to understand why Bailey's book resulted in the reaction it did, encapsulating some of the fall-out we see even today, providing an indication as to why the media portrayal of transgender issues is often so positive. Even those who fall under the transgender umbrella themselves are subjected to campaigns of harassment that prevent any meaningful debate over what it means to be transsexual or transgender (Yardley, 2014). Activists routinely try to silence media debate around transgender issues, for example early in 2017, campaigners petitioned for the BBC to not show a documentary detailing the work and dismissal of child gender dysphoria researcher Ken Zucker (Singal, 2017).

That the media depictions of transgender issues are so uncritically positive and focused on children have the same cause, the need of the autogynephilic transsexual to receive societal and interpersonal validation for their claimed identity, which is threatened when this is characterised as a paraphilia. Dreger notes central to this is concern that treatment for autogynephilic transsexuals may even become harder to procure (Dreger, 2008). This has led to a universally widespread misunderstanding of what it actually means to be transsexual and, by extension, transgender. The idea of 'feminine essence' has been used for political purposes to subvert the scientific understanding of what lies behind transsexuality to the detriment of not just transsexuals but science itself with the result that autogynephilic transsexuals are central to the promotion of transgenderism to younger children, in spite of the two types of transsexual having little in common:

> Transsexuals who have successfully accomplished the MtF transition sometimes see themselves as mentors to younger people attempting or considering this path. They may feel that public acceptance of the feminine essence narrative will facilitate the transition for these younger individuals. For example, parents may be more accepting of a child whom they think of as a female unfortunately born with a male's body than of one whom they think of as a male erotically aroused by the idea of being female… postoperative transsexuals whose desire and attachment to being women persists as their sex drive diminishes with age may come to doubt that this desire has anything to do with eroticism… this pattern is explicable via autogynephilia.
> (Bailey & Triea, 2007)

The concept of the "transgender child" is therefore central the campaigning of transgender activism. One of the most telling admissions of this instrumentalisation in contained in an interview published on YouTube between TransYouth Family Allies executive director Kim Pearson and transgender activist Autumn Sandeen (Sandeen & Pearson, 2010) with this transcription taken from the "GenderTrender" website:

> Autumn Sandeen: "I've always said there are two groups that are going to make change in transgender legislation and the "gender identity and expression" related language in legislation. It's going to be trans youth because they take, you know, they demystify it and take the sex right out of the trans experience."
>
> Kim Pearson: "They do. They do."
>
> Sandeen: "And then, transgender veterans – or people doing service like police. But it's going to be military, veterans, police, fire, those kind of folks who are serving to send a message- especially veterans. It's hard to tell a veteran, you know, "we don't appreciate your service because you're transgender".
>
> Pearson: "Right. And it's hard to say no to kids, and the needs of kids and "keeping kids safe". And you know, "being respected in schools" and things like that. It's really hard for people to say no to that."
> (GallusMag, 2012)

Where do we go from here?

Having reached this point, we have established the existence of two types of male transsexual, the homosexual and non-homosexual transsexual who are differentiated by sexual orientation and the existence of an inwardly-directed paraphilia (autogyephilia) (Blanchard, 1985) and come to understand that the concept of "gender identity" may be historically be interpreted as relating to biological sex, social environment and culture (Stoller, 1964) and for transsexuals tied to sexual orientation (Blanchard, 2008) and (Cantor, 2011). In contemporary use is can be interpreted as an innate "feeling" (Lawrence, 2013) although this is not without ideological or philosophical objections (Reilly-Cooper, 2015) and may not be supported by empirical evidence, even when claimed (Fine, 2010). We have seen how the narratives of transgender children appear to share a commonality based on culture, which is transient (Maglaty, 2011), and particularly for girls, sexual orientation. We have seen that the cross-sex identification of children often desists, with the child growing up into a homosexual adult (Cantor, 2016). We have also seen that some narratives of transgender individuals who were not "transgender children" prima facie appear influenced by pornography (Williams, 2016) and sexual fantasy (Roche, 2016). It should be abundantly clear from this analysis that the feminine pre-homosexual "trans kids" have markedly different lives and lived experiences from the non-homosexual transsexual (Blanchard, 2008) (Bailey & Triea, 2007) and that concerns expressed that the transition of children will deplete the lesbian and gay population be taken seriously, based on the evidence we have seen around sexual orientation (Gerlich, 2017).

I would suggest that any treatment protocol for children be evidence-based and dependent upon an agreed etiology for transsexualism. The present situation where the scientific enquiry and reporting of this is tightly politically controlled, in particular the attacking of any activity that is seen as being anything other than affirmative, is completely unacceptable and we should be able to have meaningful and rigorous enquiry on what it is that makes individuals 'identify' as the opposite sex. Within this field, scientific enquiry should no longer be obstructed and the routine harassment, vilification and intimidation of professionals within the field cease so that research is able to be conducted without personal or professional risk to those conducting such work, who should be free to investigate areas that at the moment would prove politically sensitive including for example investigating links between pornography consumption and autoynephilia, and childhood desistance rates. This of course can happen only with significant cultural change, especially from the transgender communities themselves.

Such cultural change can only happen if we are honest about what we already know about the etiology of transsexualism. That female and male transsexuals are different needs to be recognised and accepted, and that there are two types of male transsexual differentiated by sexual orientation needs also to be acknowledged and accepted. This in particular will require honesty from the majority of male transsexuals, those who are autogynephilic, and will require major cultural change and support from the professionals who help these people, so that the process is centred on destigmatising the truth about the subject's paraphilic sexual orientation and facilitating their coming to terms with this, rather than skirting round the issue. Such change can only happen if this is reflected in culture exogenous to the trans community, and be compassionate to these transsexuals while also addressing the myths that exist in popular culture around transsexualism. The best people to lead and motivate such a dramatic yet sensitive change would, of course, be transsexuals themselves and they should be supported by a system that allows them to live the lives they wish with access to treatments, particularly psychiatric care and therapy that is based not upon validation of cross-sex identity but to helping the patient become comfortable within their own body; any treatment that permanently alters the body should be a last resort.

Finally, we should be accepting our children for whomever and whatever they are. Biological sex should not be a barrier to children enjoying the things that they do; if our boys love pink or our girls love trucks, the response should not be to suggest their personality is incongruent with their bodies, rather that the rules we have for boys and girls need to accommodate children who do not conform to gender-based stereotypes. As gender itself is based upon stereotypes, instead of protecting concepts of "gender identity" we should protect gender non-conformity, this would have the benefit of protecting homosexuality and our homosexual children, in particular not subjecting them to a culture that threatens gender non-confirming children and adults with homophobic abuse. Finally, more and better research needs to be conducted into avenues of desistence and non-interventional options exhausted before committing any young adult to any form of medical intervention.

References

Albert, A. (2015) *Transgender children: 'I first realised Jackie was different when she was 18 months old'*. Online https://www.daynurseries.co.uk/news/article.cfm/id/1571947/Transgender-children-How-nurseries-can-support-those-with-gender-identity-issues Accessed 13 February 2017

Bailey, J. M., (2003) *The Man Who Would Be Queen: The Science of Gender-Bending and Transsexualism*. Joseph Henry Press

Bailey, J. M. &. Triea, K. (2007). What many transgender activists don't want you to know: and why you should know it anyway. *Perspectives in Biology and Medicine,* Autumn.pp. 521-534

Blanchard, R. (1985) Typology of male-to-female transsexualism. *Archives of Sexual Behaviour,* June, Volume Jun;14(3), pp. 247-61

—. (1989) The classification and labeling of nonhomosexual gender dysphorias. *Archives of Sexual Behaviour,* pp. 18, 315–334

—. (1991) Clinical observations and systematic studies of autogynephilia. *Journal of Sex and Marital Therapy,* pp. 17: 235-251

—. (1993) Partial versus complete autogynephilia and gender dysphoria. *Journal of Sex and Marital Therapy,* pp. 19: 301-307

—. (2003) *Theoretical and clinical parallels between body integrity identity disorder and gender identity disorder.* Columbia

—. (2005) Early history of the concept of autogynephilia. *Archives of Sexual Behaviour,* pp. 439-446

—. (2008) Deconstructing the feminine essence narrative.. *Archives of Sexual Behavior,* 27 June.pp. 505-10

Buhrich, N. &. M. N. (1978) Two clinically discrete syndromes of transsexualism. *British Journal of Psychiatry,* pp. Jul;133 p73-6

Butler, J. (1986) Sex and Gender in Simone de Beauvoire's Second Sex. *Yale French Studies 72,* pp. 35-49

Cantor, J. (2011) New MRI Studies Support the Blanchard Typology of Male-to-Female Transsexualism. *Archives of Sexual Behaviour,* pp. 863-864

—. (2016) *Do trans- kids stay trans- when they grow up?* http://www.sexologytoday.org/2016/01/do-trans-kids-stay-trans-when-they-grow_99.html Accessed 15 February 2017

Council, B. P. (2015) *UK Organisations Unite Against Conversion Therapy / solidarity with like-minded organisations in the USA* https://www.bpc.org.uk/news/uk-organisations-unite-against-conversion-therapy-solidarity-minded-organisations-usa_Accessed 06 07 2017 de Beauvoir, S. (1949) *Le Deuxième Sexe [The Second Sex].* Paris: Gallimard

Dreger, A. D. (2008) "The Controversy Surrounding The Man Who Would Be Queen: A Case History of the Politics of Science, Identity, and Sex in the Internet Age". *Archives of Sexual Behaviour,* Jun.p. 37(3): 366–421

—. (2015) *Answers to Some Questions about Autogynephilia.* http://alicedreger.com/autogyn Accessed 14 February 2017

Egan, N. (2016) *17 Signs I Was Transgender But Didn't Know It.* http://www.trans.cafe/posts/2016/6/27/17-signs-i-was-transgender-but-didnt-know-it Accessed 14 February 2017

Fine, C. (2010) *Delusions of Gender: How Our Minds, Society, and Neurosexism Create Difference.* Norton & Company

GallusMag (2012) *Transgender Children: "The Transgender Taboo is a Threat to Academic Freedom'.* https://gendertrender.wordpress.com/2012/01/26/transgender-children-the-transgender-taboo-is-a-threat-to-academic-freedom Accessed 9 February 2017

Gender Spectrum (2016) *Understanding Gender* https://www.genderspectrum.org/quick-links/understanding-gender Accessed 14 February 2017

Gerlich, R. (2017) *How do you know if you're "transphobic", and what is to be done about it?* https://reneejg.net/2017/02/27/how-do-you-know-if-youre-transphobic-and-what-is-to-be-done-about-it Accessed 1 March 2017

Hirshfeld, M. (1918) *Sexualpathologie Teil II 1918.* Bonn: Marcus & Weber

Kohut, R. (1972) Thoughts on narcissism and narcissistic rage. *Psychoanalytic Study of the Child,* pp. 27, 360–400

Lawrence, A. (2003) Becoming What We Love. *Perspectives in Biology and Medicine,* p. Vol 50, No4; 506–20

—. (2004) Autogynephilia: A Paraphilic Model of Gender Identity Disorder. *Journal of Gay & Lesbian Psychotherapy,* pp. 8(1/2), 69-87

—. (2008) Shame and Narcissistic Rage in Autogynephilic Transsexualism. *Arcives of Sexual Behaviour,* 23 April.p. 37:457–461

—. (2013) *Men Trapped in Men's Bodies: Narratives of Autogynephilic Transsexualism.* Springer Science & Business Media

—. (2017) Autogynephilia and the Typology of Male-to-Female Transsexualism. *European Psychologist 22(1),* pp. 39-54

Lees, P. (2014) *Kellie Maloney has always been female.* http://www.independent.co.uk/voices/comment/gender-can-t-be-bent-kellie-maloney-always-was-female-9662916.html Accessed 14 February 2017

—. (2015) *Caitlyn Jenner: a life-affirming, provocative and downright fabulous Vanity Fair cover.* https://www.theguardian.com/tv-and-radio/2015/jun/01/caitlyn-jenner-vanity-fair-cover-life-affirming Accessed 14 February 2017

Maglaty, J. (2011) *When Did Girls Start Wearing Pink?* http://www.smithsonianmag.com/arts-culture/when-did-girls-start-wearing-pink-1370097/ Accessed 14 February 2017

Moser, C. (2009) Autogynephilia in Women. *Journal of Homosexuality,* pp. 539-547

N,B.N & M. (1979) Three clinically discrete categories of fetishistic transvestism. *Archives of Sexual Behaviour ,* pp. Volume 8, Number 2

NHS Choices (2009) *My Trans Daughter* http://www.nhs.uk/Livewell/Transhealth/Pages/Transrealstorymother.aspx Accessed 14 February 2017

Price, M. (2013) *Convenience Samples: What they are, and what they should (and should not) be used for.* https://hrdag.org/2013/04/05/convenience-samples-what-they-are/ Accessed 14 February 2017

Rametti, G. et al., (2010) The microstructure of white matter in male to female transsexuals before cross-sex hormonal treatment: A DTI Study. *Journal of Psychiatric Research*

Reddit.com (2016) */r/asktransgender* https://www.reddit.com/r/asktransgender/comments/303ymf/question_about_porn/ Accessed 14 February 2017

Reilly-Cooper, R. (2015) *Sex and Gender: A Beginner's Guide.* https://sexandgenderintro.com/trans-issues-and-gender-identity Accessed 14 February 2017

Roche, J. (2016) *Other Lands.* https://thequeerness.com/2016/08/01/other-lands/ Accessed 14 February 2017

Sandeen, A. & Pearson, K. (2010) *CTLS: Interview With TransYouth Family Allies Executive Director Kim Pearson.* https://youtu.be/_b_xQzP_jHk?t=414 Accessed 14 February 2017

Savic, I. & Arver, S. (2010) Sex dimorphism of the brain in male-to-female transsexuals.. *Cerebral Cortex*

Serano, J. (2007) *Whipping Girl: A Transsexual Woman on Sexism and the Scapegoating of Feminity.* Seal Press

—. (2015) *Reconceptualizing "Autogynephilia" as Female/Feminine Embodiment Fantasies (FEFs)*. http://juliaserano.blogspot.co.uk/2015/05/reconceptualizing-autogynephilia-as_26.html Accessed 14 February 2017

Singal, J. (2017) *You Should Watch the BBC's Controversial Documentary on the Gender-Dysphoria Researcher Kenneth Zucker* http://nymag.com/scienceofus/2017/01/you-should-watch-the-bbcs-kenneth-zucker-documentary.html Accessed 14 February 2017

Stoller, R. J. (1964) A Contribution to the Study of Gender Identity. *Journal of Psychoanalysis,* pp. 220-226

—. (1968) *Sex and Gender: On the development of masculinity and femininity.* New York: Science House

Tavistock and Portman NHS Foundation Trust (2016) (2) *Gender Identity Development Service (GIDS).* https://tavistockandportman.nhs.uk/care-and-treatment/our-clinical-services/gender-identity-development-service-gids/ Accessed 14 February 2017

Tavistock and Portman NHS Foundation Trust (2016) (3) *Why Do I Feel This Way?* http://gids.nhs.uk/young-people#why-do-I-feel-this-way?#why-do-i-feel-this-way Accessed 14 February 2017

—. (2016) (4) *Gender Identity and Sexuality.* http://gids.nhs.uk/gender-identity-and-sexuality Accessed 14 February 2017

—. (2016) *Gender Identity Development Service Statistics* https://tavistockandportman.nhs.uk/documents/408/gids-service-statistics.pdf Accessed 14 February 2017

Williams, R. (2016) *Autogynephilia - A Critique and Personal Narrative.* [Online] Available at: http://www.philpercs.com/2016/02/autogynephilia-a-critique-and-personal-narrative.html Accessed 14 February 2017

World Health Organisation (undated) *'What do we mean by "sex" and "gender"?* http://apps.who.int/gender/whatisgender/en/ Accessed 14 February 2017

Yardley, M. (2014) *Kellie Maloney, Newsnight and the debate the transgender community refused to have.* http://www.newstatesman.com/politics/2014/08/kellie-maloney-newsnight-and-debate-transgender-community-refused-have Accessed 14 February 2017

—. (2015) *What Does It Mean to be Caitlyn?* https://www.morningstaronline.co.uk/a-d78a-What-does-it-mean-to-be-Caitlyn#.WKWT6_nyjIU Accessed 14 February 2017

—. (2017) *Common Threads And Narratives of Transgender Children And What This Means For Our Lesbian And Gay Populations.* http://mirandayardley.com/en/common-threads-and-narratives-of-transgender-children-and-what-this-means-for-our-lesbian-and-gay-populations/

CHAPTER NINE

UNHEARD VOICES OF DETRANSITIONERS

CAREY MARIA CATT CALLAHAN

In this chapter, I will trace the emergence of a new kind of womanhood - women returned from trans identity. Like many births, it happened in a rush. Very quickly, almost all at once, it was the same thought in several women's heads, then it was a group formed in Oakland, California, then it was many women reading each other's writing, creating online forums, compiling stories, designing surveys, planning meetings, strategizing on delivering support to the wave of women joining us. This chapter must necessarily zoom into the crevices of my individual story and pan out to ideological narratives that rule our culture. Realizing you were enabled in a ritual divorce from the female body and then choosing, despite all cultural pressure, to return, feels something like splitting the atom- the fundamentals of a shared social reality shift, and unknown potentials loom, both grand and ominous. Ideologies which had operated invisibly are now stark and unavoidable in their visibility.

It took until I was detransitioned before I noticed all the statues of women in downtown Cleveland weren't of real women. I don't mean the bodies portrayed weren't sufficiently curvy to carry a Dove soap campaign. I mean none of the statues represent women who lived on this earth at any point in time. They are instead statues of women who signify concepts: the spirit of the city, the muse of scientific knowledge, the goddesses of industry and progress. Then there is a statue of Jesse Owens, who won four gold medals at the Berlin Olympics in 1936, Alexander Hamilton, who authored the Federalist Papers and another of General Moses Cleaveland, who founded the city.

The statues of women have figures that aren't as emaciated as current beauty culture would prefer. They are "real" in the contemporary use of that word- the bellies are not concave, the upper arms have both biceps and triceps. If anything the heft in the arms and thighs is comfortingly reminiscent of my bulk. These giantesses sit in robes, holding scrolls and tablets, gazing pensively over downtown as if it were their salon.

They are female bodies. They aren't people. They're concepts. The female body is lovely to gaze upon, and since we like these concepts, we make the concepts lovely female bodies.

The male body is not so lovely to gaze upon. I myself like to gaze upon them, but it would be unseemly to decorate public space with many highly gaze-able male forms. You wouldn't just sculpt a huge bronze male body and stick it downtown unless it looked like a person who had done something you wanted to remember. Men do things worthy of remembering. Somehow this public invisibility was lost on me in my lust to inhabit a male form. I did fantasize about testosterone aiding me in developing a shredded physique, and yet more than that I wanted to not represent a thing. To just be, my form calling forth no meaning besides the specifics of who I was and what I accomplished.

When I was deeper into being trans, after a course of testosterone but financially delayed in obtaining my mastectomy, I went over a new friend's house in San Francisco. I lived in Oakland, and didn't understand the busses in San Francisco, so everywhere I went had to be in working distance of the BART train line. This new friend was a trans man. His house was barely within walking distance of a BART stop- it was up a hill and the last three blocks were steep enough to mimic the burning thighs of Stairmaster-ing. It was worth it to me to get to his house. I was having a lot of trouble being trans. I did not feel the way I thought I was going to. Being a woman had felt like I walked through the world with a billboard in front of my face, advertising a product I didn't have in stock. The product was motherly, sexually available, kind, nurturing. Being a trans man quite surprisingly felt similar. What was on the billboard was harder for me to parse- still sexually available, still open to unpaid emotional labour, but interested in broadly male experiences- weight-lifting, strip clubs and power tools. The product on the billboard was slightly different, but still one I didn't have to sell. I had expected the billboard to fall away. I had expected the feeling of performance to go away. The social expectations of performing "trans man" were not so different from the social expectations of performing "woman." I had naively expected transitioning would enable me to navigate the world without performance.

Saying this feeling out loud was worth the burn in my thighs. I got to his co-op house, populated by progressive people from moneyed families, and we sat in a lush backyard garden. He was the result of a friend set up- my radical queer friends from Chicago knew I was having a rough go of it with transition, and thought another trans man would talk me through it. He had transitioned young, in the first two years at his women's college, and now at 28 passed as a baby-faced man. He seemed to relish the contradictions between the billboard and the person behind it. He was in a writing seminar with a famous lesbian poet who wanted him to write about his mother, and he said he was happy to. His lineage in the lesbian tradition and its tension with his male identification seemed something like an interesting puzzle to keep on his desk at work- pick it up, play with it, set it down when he had better things to do. The tensions between my billboard and the me that was carrying it were wearing me down to the nub. The class stuff, the sex stuff, the stereotype stuff, and especially the emotional work I knew was not being asked of male men- whatever mysterious this new billboard advertised I was tired of its weight. I had simply wanted to live without a billboard.

 I told him a version of this. I told him my breasts were only getting harder to have on my body, that my thighs were only torturing me more with their existence, that my daily feelings of wanting to tear parts of me off myself was only more pronounced as the result of social transition. I told him the social role of trans man was not the manhood I had fantasized about all these years. I said I was sick to death of other people's eyes. I said I wondered who I would be without people's eyes on me. "Ah yes, I've thought about that a lot," he replied. "What gender would I be in the wilderness, with only the birds flying overhead to see me?"

 That sounded like the right world for me. Me and the birds - who would never use a pronoun for me. Without other people's eyes, I wouldn't be anything more than a moving body, legs that propelled me forward, arms that picked up detritus one eats in the woods. My new friend seemed at ease with the nascent implication of the scenario- the problem wasn't my breasts and thighs, it was other people's eyes on my breasts and thighs. The birds wouldn't be interested in those parts of mine. Those parts wouldn't speak over the whole. He had had some of those parts removed. It was because we don't live in those woods. Other people's eyes land on us from all directions.

 This is what happens when female people talk to each other, even when they have made very different choices, even when one is at peace with a path that is killing the other. When female people speak one on one, the moving parts are identified, the implications are highlighted. When female people speak to each other it is as if the statues in downtown Cleveland have turned their face towards each other, whispering what they know about who is running who around the city streets, making plans for how to finally lift their heft. When women step out of their frozen forms, turn our faces to each other, we can whisper the stories of how we were sculpted:

> "I didn't see any way I could be a woman. I saw how different others treated me when they thought I was a boy, when they were unable to see me as female because they never learned a face, body, posture, voice like mine could belong to a woman. As a boy, I fit inside their world, even as a trans boy I usually made more sense, caused less confusion than as a girl. If I was a trans boy we could all agree something was wrong, my body was wrong, I had the wrong traits and character for my body but that could be fixed and then order would be restored"
> Crash, www.crashchaoscats.wordpress.com/2016/12/16/reclaiming-female speaking-back

How do you find another detransitioned woman to speak quietly to? When I finally knew that this new billboard was as suffocating as the one I grew up with, that I needed to find some way to access authenticity even with the world's unrelenting demand for a conveniently gendered presentation from me, I searched online. I emailed a listserv named "NoGoingBack," and never got a response. I told a trans woman friend of mine this, a woman I'd lent money to and talked down from suicidal threats, and she laughed. It was clear to me, regardless of an internal felt sense of gendered self, I'd done the caretaking work in the friendship and she couldn't even conceive of herself as owing me some in return. I posted on craigslist looking for someone who'd gone through the detransition experience. I got a description of someone's penis, and a couple of offers to take me out to coffee because I sounded "fascinating." I finally cried to my therapist about it, "How can I be the only one who has gotten this wrong and figured it out so late in the game?" She emailed her supervisor who emailed another therapist, and got me the pseudonym of a detransitioned woman who agreed to meet me for coffee.

    I remember she looked like a normal woman but she had the low voice from testosterone I now had. I remember we talked about dissociation that first day - how I had pieced together that my chronic sense of my body being surreal and wrong was tied to other dissociative symptoms I experienced, the intrusive sense I was living in a movie, my chronic dreaminess and distractibility, which was tied to my racing thoughts and jumpiness. I remember she speculated to me that modern society is based on a foundation of dissociation, that authenticity must be based on some loyalty to your body's experience of the world and it was almost impossible to be loyal to your body's experience and pay your rent. I remember telling her I think I got turned around from sexual trauma and the soup of sexism I had been living in. I remember her saying that was her story too.

She asked if I wanted to meet another detransitioned woman. We made another date. Then a week later there were three of us, sitting on some grass by Lake Merritt, keeping our voices low in case someone passing by heard us. What was the authority we were scared of being surveilled by? There was a pervasive sense in 2014 that what we were talking about was off-limits to say. If you brought sexism and objectification into the equation of why someone might want to transition, you were abandoning the trans community, and only bigots would do that. So we spoke low and glanced up at the people walking by to be sure they weren't paying attention to us. Then we made dinner plans to skype with a fourth detransitioned woman who lived in another state. Then we began to meet on Friday nights, to eat and talk.

If you had asked me in 2012, while I was transitioning, if a detransitioned woman existed, I would have scoffed and speculated there was probably some random, lonely lost soul like that. In 2014 I claimed the label detransitioned for myself, took on the cross of being a random, lost soul, and then quite suddenly had a weekly support group with three more women like me. In 2016 Cari, a 22-year-old detransitioned woman who blogs at http://guideonragingstars.tumblr.com, posted an online survey for detransitioned women and received 203 responses. One response is:

> When I first learned transition existed, when I was around 13, I was really intrigued, but never considered it as a possibility for myself- the cost was too high. These were people I only saw on daytime talk shows when I stayed home sick, getting called really horrible names and treated as spectacles. Over the next few years, as I gradually learned more about transition and got to know more individuals who were transitioning online, I felt less and less like transitioning would make me a freak or totally alone. By the time I was around 16, the cost/benefit equation had shifted considerably in my eyes, enough for me to start pursuing transition.
>
> In a way, it's a good thing that I didn't judge myself as harshly for having a drive to transition. I don't think people who want to transition, or who do transition, should feel like they're disgusting freaks for it, the way I used to. And of course, not transitioning alone wouldn't have resolved any of the trauma or pervasive lifelong gendered rejection that made me want to escape femaleness. It's not like I would be totally fine if I had just managed to avoid one maladaptive coping mechanism. Given that no healthier options were made accessible to me, I was going to keep trying self-preservation strategies with high costs, transition or

no transition. I might have had more serious alcohol issues, thrown myself into casual sex, whatever. Something was gonna have to give.
—Max, bornwrong.tumblr.com/2016/09/07/socialcontagion

We talked about all the ways we had hurt ourselves. Transition was only one way out of many. There were drugs, starving yourself, abusive relationships disguised as kinky ones. There were groups of "friends" who we believed it was normal to be scared of, normal to find that one day you were the one called out, and on that day it would be normal for you to lose all of your important relationships at once. There were radical queer scenes where credibility depended on sexual availability - attending the right sex parties, proving you would date or at least have sex with every gender in every kind of body. We talked about all the times we had given ourselves away trying to measure up, to prove ourselves righteous standard bearers for a radical queer politic that more than our action, more than our intelligence, more than our solidarity, demanded sexual access. We talked about desiring women when the most desirable person to be was a female who refused to go by that name. We talked about the disorientation of finding we'd been had - that the feminism you'd come to for liberation would let you call yourself any pronoun you wanted, but like every other social group on the planet, your value depended on your willingness to play mother and hooker.

I wasn't sure I wanted to call myself a feminist anymore. It seemed calling yourself one was a setup to be accused of not being good enough to be one. I was tired of other people getting to tell me if I was good enough. I wanted to be more precious to myself than being good. I wanted to rest and heal. I wanted to feel like my body was real and correct. I wanted to lose the sensation of being watched all the time. So I wrote, and my detransitioned friends wrote. For my pseudonym I chose my two middle names. My father had, in the immediate aftermath of birth, given me the middle name "Maria" as homage to my midwife. My mother, upon awakening, had insisted on "Catt" as homage to Carrie Chapman Catt, the American suffragette. Using my middle names reflected the project behind my writing. I wanted to know who I was at my core, deep in the middle of who I was, behind the facades I had invested in. My friends and I hid behind pseudonyms and we were grateful for the anonymity.

December 2009

I told one person. And then another. And then another. I started dressing the way I wanted to and cut my hair up above my ears. People knew and things changed. No one started conversations with me anymore unless they couldn't avoid it and then they'd babble awkwardly and look away like they were trying to avoid staring at something stuck in my teeth.

If I looked at a girl for longer than a couple of seconds or smiled at a girl in the hallway or was too friendly when I had to talk to another girl in class, her inevitable reaction was some mixture of fear and disgust. Whenever it happened I remembered how I'd felt about Jacob trying to force his sweaty palm into my hand. I wondered if she felt the same way about me.

I avoided going to the bathroom at school as much as possible. When I had to, I looked to make sure no one was watching before I opened the door and prayed no one would be inside when I got in. I knew someone might perceive a boy slipping into the wrong bathroom and I knew no straight girl would want to be alone in there with me.

I heard "is that a boy or a girl?" often. People didn't bother to lower their voices. I felt disgusting. I felt wrong. The person everyone was seeing when they looked at me wasn't me. I didn't want to be the dyke they thought I was anymore. I didn't even want to be in my body anymore.

June 2010

I told everyone to start calling me Daniel and 'he' instead of 'she'. I make a plan to go to a new school in the fall where everyone will think I'm a normal boy. I'll be able to blend in. No one will see a weird, dishevelled, dangerous lesbian when they look at me anymore. I think everything is going to be okay now. - desisterressister.tumblr.com/2017/01/03/how alesbianbecameatransboy

In the beginning my grief was about the loss of my sustaining dream. In the beginning the harm that had been done to me because of my female body came rushing back, and the hopeful split vanished: the possibility that perhaps my female body was not the real me. Perhaps in some important way I had not been in the room when I was hurt, perhaps there was no malice but simply a misunderstanding of my gender. Perhaps that had not been my real life: all that hopeful, comforting rupture slipped away. I was simply a cast aside, crazy woman: a crazy woman like all the other pathetic women who had been tortured to psychosis throughout the centuries. In the beginning my grief was a howl for the time, the money, the space in my own head I given to a dream that was never going to be mine.

I healed. It was as slow as tectonic drift. I prayed a lot because I wasn't sure if I was a crazy person or not and I wasn't sure if I could put my life back together. I went to a lot of yoga. I shot lasers at the facial hair that I had grown. I learned about contouring and dry shampoo. Eventually I knew, because the face looking back at me in the mirror looked so unremarkable, that I would be fine, that the past was the past. That with enough distance and a long enough ponytail I would not be accused of being a different kind of trans person, That with enough distance and the mastering of mascara I would be forgiven this episode. I would write my anonymous blog I would read other women's anonymous blogs I would be normal and contemplate that unfortunate period behind closed doors, as a private endeavour.

Except my private endeavour was connecting me to women who were quite young, and who had been subject to more medical interventions than I had gotten - longer courses of testosterone, mastectomies. So they position this treatment as the One And Only and, shove us away and onto it and then don't even research the effects of what they're giving us. A quick glance over the Society of General Internal Medicine's 2014 Cancer Risk and Prevention in Transgender Patients makes it clear, repeatedly, how little we know (or at least how little we knew just two years ago): "MTF individuals receiving feminizing hormones experience breast cancer, yet the degree of risk relative to natal females is uncertain." "There are no long-term studies on endometrial cancer incidence among FTM individuals." "No long-term studies have investigated ovarian cancer incidence among FTM individuals." We don't know. We don't know. We don't know. Or maybe, we don't care. We don't care. We don't care. Resisterdesister.tumblr.com/2016/10/27/Themedicalcommunityisfailinggenderdysphoricpeople

Many of us tell half-truths and live by obscured vision, seeing just enough to survive. There is no way to live without some contact and knowledge of how reality actually runs. The whole organism knows, even if parts of it, the parts that interpret and make meaning of sensations consciously, pretend to know something different. The organism does what it needs to do to survive and if this means knowing exactly what's going on and lying about it at the same time, so be it. But such a life is lived in tension and is another stress upon the life force it would rather do without. So it accepts this for the sake of survival but it seeks at the same time to bring the pieces back together into wholeness, bring it all back into knowledge and sensation. Many people are selves at war with their organism, mirroring on a small scale the warfare of the larger world. Crash, https://crashchaoscats. wordpress.com/2016/12/16/reclaiming-femalespeaking-back/#more-839

In 2016 Cari wrote a survey for detransitioned women that received 203 responses. Those responses showed the average age for transition for females who would go on to detransition was 17 years. The responses showed the average age of detransition was 21 years. Cari asked survey respondents to comment on how they felt about transition's role in their own lives. The responses were far from homogenous. It was clear there were many different meanings to be made of pursuing medical interventions to affirm a gender identity that had since shifted or vanished:

> "Wish I didn't have to go through all that confusion and obsession."

> "I was in a bad mental health place and dealing with a pretty severe eating disorder. Transition helped me kind of "recover," so I can't feel totally negative about it. But I regret it and wish I'd been able to recover another way."

> "I don't really regret it. Going through it forced me to become a braver, more confident person, and I like most of the permanent changes to my body too (voice, body hair, clit size). I had some awful experiences in the trans community and I'm bitter about the way I was treated, and way I treated others, due to ideology. But if I hadn't transitioned, , I don't think I could have ever reached the place I am now, where I'm actually pleased and proud to be a woman in spite of everything."

> "I used transition as self-harm. It destroyed so many parts of my life."

> "I have major body issues due to the effects of T and my mental health was wrecked by stealth."

> "I don't regret physical transition, but I think identity politics are dumb."

> "It felt pointless, nothing changed and nothing improved. The only thing that happened was my resentment at being female being enabled."

> "My body is mine, even with the beard, chest hair, etc. I have nothing to be ashamed of."

Stella, Cari (2016) "Female Detransition and Reidentification: Survey results and interpretation"
http://guideonragingstars.tumblr.com/post/149877706175/female-detransition-and-reidentification-survey

These responses show the multiplicity of viewpoints detransitioned women hold regarding the modifications they made to their bodies and their experience of socially separating themselves from being viewed as women. Some respondents to the survey found the construct of a non-binary identity helpful to their understanding of themselves. When other people refer to me using "they' pronouns and speculate I am non-binary or genderqueer I reflexively close my eyes and shake at disgust at the notion. For me being set apart from other female people in that manner reminds me of the fetishistic sexual attention I often received while I was trans identified and so I'm done with gender identity thank you very much. But reading the survey results was a lesson in multiplicity: an experience that looks so similar creates such different insights and emotions.

Emotional states are generally not permanent, and our assessments of experiences in our lives are similarly in flux. My assessment of my choice to detransition at 32 years of age was much different than my assessment two years later. At 32 I thought, *"I have to investigate the chance there's another way to approach these feelings besides making them my identity because I'm so close to killing myself on this path."* At 34 I think *"Wow, these feelings that used to run my life have receded into red flags that alert me to when my daily anxiety levels have been too high for too long."* I sometimes catch myself in the mirror and wish my breasts were gone. These days I am just as likely to look in the mirror and appreciate how unlike a magazine image my naked body looks. In a world that seeks to narrow the range of what females look like, my body resists of its own accord, regardless of the inner critic. My thoughts capitulate to the tyranny of capitalist images much more than my body feels the need to:

> Is transition a selfish act? Insofar as any acts intended to be self-preserving over all else are, yeah. It's worth noting here that the perception of attempted self-preservation as immorally selfish is applied very sparingly to the actions of white, straight men, but broadly applied to anyone female (especially women dehumanized in additional ways), even by other women within feminist community. Are we entitled to protect our own lives to the best of our ability, or aren't we? Under patriarchy, women are frequently presented with situations in which it is not in their own immediate best interests to act out feminist principles. Shitting on FTMs is not any more politically justifiable than mocking a woman for wearing makeup to work or getting "feminizing" cosmetic surgery. I absolutely do not believe that transition is more selfish than expecting other women to self-flagellate for having transitioned. Condemning someone for choosing (under duress!) an option that kept

her alive but did not uplift other women is not compatible with a realistic assessment of the threats women live under.
—Max, bornwrong.tumblr.com/2016/10/118/strategy

What do the voices of detransitioned women say? As our presence and the spectrum of our writing expand the themes we explore refuse to participate in hyperbole. We say our bodies deserve love. We say we struggle to provide that love. We say the blame rests on lesbophobia and a queer theory which glamorizes disembodiment. We say the blame rests on personal mental illness. We say it was a crime what was done to us. We say other people's choices can't be up to us:

> I felt I had no choice but transition for a long time, and the reason I felt that way was because other choices were not offered to me. I didn't know anyone who had survived feelings like mine without transition, and I didn't have any ideas about how someone might do that. That's a problem! How can someone give informed consent to transition when they believe the only alternative is a miserable life eventually cut short by suicide? People who transition believing it's absolutely the only way they can ever experience any relief are people whose community and healthcare professionals have failed them.
> —Max, bornwrong.tumblr.com/22017/01/04/choice

> As I've gotten older I've found tremendous relief from learning not to let dysphoria in or indulge it as a means of validating my gender identity. I've also found tremendous relief from processing all of the lesbophobia and misogyny I'd internalized. Mindfulness and exercise have also been a help. I've grown. I've learned to live in this body. I've learned to love myself as a lesbian. But fifteen-year-old me, sitting trembling and scared in my gender therapist's office for the first time, didn't know that that was possible. My therapist certainly didn't ever tell me it was. Once she'd determined that my dysphoria was real (and, god, was it real,) there was one path. It involved turning my life upside down to go "stealth," taking testosterone and eventually surgical intervention. I made it through the first two steps before I started to figure out there was another way.
> —Hailey www.desisterresister.wordpress.com/2016/10/27/the-medical-community-is-failin g-dysphoric-people/

In January 2011 another online survey of detransitioned women carried out by the blogger Re-Sister, taught us more about the psychological context of inappropriate transition. Re-Sister received 211 replies from detransitioned women detailing the co-morbid diagnoses and suspected psychological conditions of the cohort. She also asked *"Do you feel that any of the conditions listed above contributed to your trans identification and/or transition? If so, how?"* Some replies she received:

> "Feeling foreign in my body from a young age due to sensory issues, bullying, and emotional abuse definitely all played a role in my uncertainty of my gender identity. I didn't want to associate with the horrors of being a woman abused from the get-go, so I tried to opt out mentally"

> "The ASD makes my social understanding of gender very abstract, and it also leads me to feel out of place, and that if I was ungendered I wouldn't have many of the problems I have."

> "Dissociation was a way to escape from the problems I was experiencing. I did not like the person I was and assuming a trans identity made me feel better for a few years. I had severe depression because I was a lesbian and gender nonconforming,
>
> I think it was easier for me to accept being trans and straight rather than homosexual and gender non-conforming"

> "Borderline personality disorder's unstable sense of self contributed to it I think"

> "When my PTSD and BPD were at their worst, I had no sense of self but I knew I didn't want to be a woman because bad things happen to women. I developed a very masculine self at a young age after being raped, and it was absolutely to dissociate myself from the pain. Once I started receiving psychological and psychiatric help, started therapy and started taking medication for my conditions, I began to discover and create my true self and realized that my masculine "armor" was a harmful coping mechanism I had developed in order to avoid my very real problems. I am now a happier femme lesbian."

> "Probably not. I think I had been so many times that cis women 'identify' as women and I just... didn't. I thought my experience of gender was different from that of a woman. I had 'social' dysphoria ie I didn't like being seen as/treated like a woman. I had dysphoria around my breasts because they are so female and sexualized. I felt like my attraction to women was a very masculine trait."

> "No. I believe my anxiety is comorbid with my transsexualism but did not create it."

> "I think autism had something to do with my childhood difficulties relating to other girls and understanding/performing femininity. Traits

like difficulty socialising, extreme focus on very specific interests etc seemed more acceptable once I framed myself as a boy."

The results of Re-Sister's survey can be found at www.desister resister.files.wordpress.com/2017/01/survey-1.pdf. Every reply to her open-ended question about the relationship of co-morbid diagnoses to the creation of a trans identity can be found at www.desisterresister. files.wordpress.com/2017/01/data_q8_161204.pdf.

Reading the replies to Re-Sister's survey is to take in the full picture of how we are failing young women. Young women trying to make sense of why their patterns of thought seem different from other women, why they can't function in the same way, why they can't perform femininity, why they are compulsive, why their bodies don't feel real, why they return to feeling sad again and again. Feminism now offers the narrative that if you feel uncomfortable with the stereotypes projected onto members of your sex, your gender identity is the likely culprit. Kate Bornstein's *"My Gender Workbook"* Janet Mock's *"Redefining Realness"* writings by Ivan E. Coyote, Pat Califia, Jennifer Finney Boylan and more frame gender transition as a transgressive pursuit of individual authenticity, while leave out of the story of that pursuit the power relationships attendant with disciplining the body through pharmacology.

    I wonder what kind of feminism would have led me to choices that prioritized my bodily health. I wonder what kind of feminism would have located my locus of identity not on the self as presented to others, but on the roaming witness that wakes up each morning to make sense of the world. I wonder what kind of feminism would have given me support for my own mental health struggles, would have told me that anxiety, depression, PTSD only made me more valuable, rather than a burden or an embarrassment. I wonder what kind of feminism would have created space for all the ways I needed help, rather than extolling an ethic of strength and exceptionalism that added to my feelings of shame and failure. I wonder what kind of feminism can create space for brains and bodies that society has to label "masculine," to invisibilize the restriction and discipline necessary to produce a body and brain labelled "feminine."

    What I have found in the community of detransitioned women, more than I have experienced in any other feminist community, is a focus on taking care of the body and respecting that witness. I have found a promise that a sister's wellbeing is of more concern than the ideas currently being parsed in her head. An interest in the details of the path she walks along. A knowledge that without a multiplicity of viewpoints we cannot begin to see the moving parts that power the whole. Why wasn't this the feminism I found before detransition? Why was there a right way to look and a right way to think and a right way to date? Why was the inside of my head treated like a bowl to be filled with approved thoughts, instead of its own spring of needed knowledge?

In the fall of 2016 I got an email from a woman considering transition. She wrote that she wanted to be an explorer, to climb mountains, and it would be safer to do that in a male body. The distinction between a male body and a female body masculinized with the aid of doctors was not one she had considered.

I propose that even the most liberation focused radical feminists have forgotten to respect young women as explorers. I propose that the voices of detransitioned women matter not only as an indictment of the medical industry or of queer politic, but as a warning that young women are in too many relationships where they must maintain a proper aesthetic as symbols and not speaking, moving, seeing subjects in the world. I propose that too-often even with their loved ones they feel themselves to be treasured objects, beautiful daughters on display, rather than actors, subjects, explorers valued for the sights their eyes can see, which without their words we ourselves will never know. This is the potential I see in the 203 detransitioned women Cari gathered. A feminism that compels us to move as we wish, tells us to observe and report and tells us the object the world can judge is incidental to the subject behind the eyes.

In a world that wants us to be billboards and statues we resist flattening into symbols. In a world that wants us to signify we hold onto the world as woods. That dangerous and surprising world the body acts within and upon, the world where birds fly a thousand miles every year, where cities are founded, where governments are planned, where races are won. A world where unfortunately the objects we are judged to be must also be navigated and yet what has always mattered are the horizons our eyes can see.

Readers, as re-identified women return, bringing back the lessons, the views, the hidden ideologies they can now make out, do you have your ear turned to them? Can you relate to us not as symbols or signifiers but as explorers reporting back? Can we live in your imaginations as the researchers, writers, healers, leaders we are, rather than sitting frozen representing catastrophe or liberation? We are speaking, no longer in whispers, but at full volume.

These are the writings of detransitioned women. Please read.

crashchaoscats.wordpress.com
redressalert.tumblr.com
guideonragingstars.tumblr.com
twentythreetimes.tumblr.com
bOrnwrOng.wordpress.com
kittyit.tumblr.com
desisterresister.wordpress.com
https://hotflanks.wordpress.com
thissoftspace.wordpress.com
Blood and Visions zine Autotomous Womyn's Press available at
    http://www.greenwomanstore.com/blood-and-visions.html
www.mariacatt.com
www.careycallahan.com

Reference

Beck, Aaron, T.; Rush, A. John; Shaw, Brian F.; Emery, Gary (1987) *Cognitive Therapy of Depression.* Guilford Press

CHAPTER TEN

THE VIEW FROM THE CONSULTING ROOM

ROBERT WITHERS

What is the best way to understand and work therapeutically with someone who suffers serious discomfort because they feel their core gender identity is at odds with their biological sex? Gender reassignment surgery and hormone therapy often seem to be the treatment of choice currently. Many claim to be well satisfied with the results (see e.g. Murad et al, 2010). The accounts of detransitioners however, testify that some decidedly are not (see e.g. Blood and Visions, 2015 as well as this book). Do health professionals and trans-people owe it to themselves then, to seriously consider other ways of working before resorting to radical, irreversible and potentially harmful medical procedures? Can psychoanalytic psychotherapy offer such an alternative? Or is there a danger that thinking about gender dysphoria psychologically will add to its stigmatisation? These are the questions this chapter will be raising.

Unlike inter-sex states, there is no credible evidence of a physical component in gender dysphoria (see Dreger, 2015 and Withers, 2015). In contrast, as I hope to show, several psychological factors may help us understand it. So closing a discussion of these factors down in order to protect trans people from stigmatisation (see e.g. UKCP, 2012) seems a bit like deliberately throwing the compass overboard when we have no other way of navigating.

I attended a weekend conference called *Transgender, Gender and Psychoanalysis* at the Freud museum recently. Participants from the floor were literally shaking as they raised their questions. The fear of being accused of transphobia was palpable in the room. Even the well-known psychoanalyst Danny Nobus noted that one's subjective gender identity is discovered not chosen without daring to discuss the possible role of the unconscious in that discovery. He was still attacked. Freud could be heard turning in his grave!

It is the purpose of this chapter to open up that discussion now. What are some of the possible unconscious psychological factors underlying gender dysphoria? I realise that asking this question makes me vulnerable to accusations of transphobia. But I believe that such accusations do trans-people a disservice by discouraging them from considering alternatives to life-long hormone treatment and surgery. They also perpetuate the cultural stigmatisation of mental illness by bowing to it. That stigmatisation probably arises from a deep seated fear of our own madness (Foucault, 1961). With the publication of books such as the present one, comes the hope that the tide is finally turning as a growing number of health professionals, trans-individuals and their friends and families become willing to consider alternatives to the medicalisation of transgendered states.

This chapter is largely derived from my work at *The Rock Clinic* a busy, collectively-run, community-based, charitable psychotherapy and counselling service in Brighton. I have practiced there for over thirty years as a therapist and twenty as a supervisor. Although my training as an analyst enables me to see people up to five times a week, many prefer to work weekly, for practical reasons. With them I consider myself a psychoanalytic psychotherapist; that is a psychotherapist whose approach is informed by psychoanalysis. In practice it would be hard to distinguish that work from psychodynamic counselling.

People consult me for a wide variety of conditions. But Brighton is famous as the LGBT capital of Britain, so over the years I have seen my fair share of trans clients in various stages of transition. All case material will either be used with the express consent of the individual concerned, consist of a composite case without distinguishing features, or have been published elsewhere. All names have been changed to preserve anonymity.

In psychotherapy each relationship is unique - that is part of the work's enduring fascination- so it would be wrong to set too much store by generalisations. Gender dysphoria, like most other conditions, can arise from a variety of sources. Here though are four of the ways in which psychoanalytic thinking may be able to help us understand and hence work with it:

1) Children and adolescents who identify as trans are increasingly asking for and receiving hormones to block puberty (Di Ceglie, 2017). The hope seems to be that the alarmingly high suicide and self-harm rates (Dhejne et al, 2011 etc.) among post-operative transsexuals will be reduced if a person has not

experienced themselves in an alien, sexually adult body. It is too early to know the results of this experiment. But from my perspective as a psychoanalytic psychotherapist, the impulse to block puberty in this way seems far from neutral. It can be symptomatic, for instance, of a fear of adult sexuality. A similar refusal of adult sexuality can underlie adolescent anorexia, where it may have fatal consequences. As with anorexia (Orbach, 1978), there may be ways of tackling this fear psychotherapeutically.

2) It is possible to think of many trans-people as identifying with a mind of one gender while dissociating powerfully from their oppositely gendered body (Withers, 2015). Psychoanalysis provides an account of how, in health, a person comes to feel at home in their own body (Winnicott, 1949). It goes on to describe how trauma and deprivation can disrupt this process leading to *mind-body dissociation* (Winnicott 1949, 1964). Analytic practice [see e.g. Winnicott (1949, 1963) and Ogden (2001)] opens up potential ways of working with this feature of transgendered experience psychotherapeutically.

3) From Freud on, psychoanalysis has regarded us all as psychologically part-male and part-female (Freud, 1905 Jung, 1951a etc.). In health these elements can interact creatively (Freud 1916, Jung 1951a, Britton, 1989). Sometimes however a powerful *dissociation* develops between male and female elements in the personality and then gender dysphoria may be experienced (Winnicott, 1966, Jung, 1951b). When it is, analytic thinking may be able open up ways of both understanding and working therapeutically with it (Winnicott, 1966).

4) Psychoanalysis can furnish us with an account of how our sense of self emerges from interactions and identifications with people in our environment (BPSG, 2010). In this way it can help us understand how a person may come to feel identified with one part of themselves but disgusted by another disowned part (Orbach, 2009). This may manifest as disgust with part of one's own body. In my experience this is something trans-individuals often feel. *Identification* can also act as a substitute for the emotional work involved in mourning (Freud, 1917). A person can sometimes 'become' someone else in unconscious fantasy, rather than grieving the loss of that person emotionally.

This too has implications for working psychotherapeutically with certain trans-individuals (Di Ceglie, 2009).

I will be arguing that psychoanalysis has the potential to contribute to our understanding of, and therapeutic work with, individuals who identify as trans or gender dysphoric in all these ways. But first it will be necessary to pause to anticipate some potential objections to this project.

Some possible grounds for objection

Psychoanalysis has come in for some fierce and sustained criticism over the years. It is not evidence based (Eysenck, 1985), it is 'mother blaming' (ibid.), Freud was sexually obsessed, Jung a mystic; and so on. Despite such widespread hostility, psychoanalysis and its derivatives (psychodynamic counselling and psychoanalytic psychotherapy) seem to continue to play an influential role in Western culture, given the proliferation of courses, conferences, publications, therapists and their clients associated with the field . Considerations of space only allow me to focus on possible grounds for specific objections to the current project, rather than address such general doubts and criticisms. But I will briefly return to the issue of mother blaming later in the chapter.

Conversion therapy?

Historically psychoanalysis, like society in general, has to its shame, pathologised homosexuality. These days attempts to 'cure' people of their homosexuality are rightly outlawed (UKCP, 2012). But isn't there a danger that seeking an analytic understanding of trans-phenomena could encourage similar attempts to 'cure' people of being trans?

The Canadian psychologist Ken Zucker was recently suspended from work and his Toronto gender identity clinic closed down following such allegations, which he denies. Zucker was the subject of a recent BBC documentary *Transgender Kids: Who Knows Best* which in my opinion gave a very balanced view of the issues involved. Zucker's main point is very simple. Gender identity in adolescence is not stable. So offering people irreversible medical treatment then is a mistake. Most will grow out of their cross-sex identification quite naturally and after a period of experimentation are quite likely to become happily gay, bi-sexual, gender fluid or even straight. He also points out that adolescents with autistic traits sometimes self-identify as trans. Help with their autism would be more appropriate than irreversible medical treatment for them too.

Zucker seems to me to be practicing common sense rather that conversion therapy here. In fact those advocating earlier access to hormones and surgery could themselves be accused of effectively advocating gay conversion therapy. But I do not know all the details of Zucker's case, so do not feel qualified to comment further on it. What I do know is that psychoanalysis has tried to learn from its previous pathologisation of homosexuality (see e.g. Denman in Withers, 2003). So it is unlikely that any competent psychoanalytic psychotherapist would hold a trans-conversion agenda; at least consciously. The idea of helping a person become themselves more effectively is central to all schools of analytic therapy. For the transgendered person, this might mean finding ways of living creatively with their gender fluidity even if that challenges current cultural and family norms. I would argue that it is the attempt to physically alter one's body to comply with a conscious mental picture of oneself that reinforces current 'gender-binary' cultural rigidity; not psychoanalysis. So while psychoanalytic therapy might try to help a person live more comfortably with their gender dysphoria, only turning to surgery as a last resort, it would be hard to argue that this is an attempt to 'cure' them of being trans. Nevertheless therapists do have an unconscious which is bound to impact upon their work. I will be arguing that it is crucial for the therapist (as well as their clients) to be able to acknowledge and work with this; especially their own 'mad' parts. The therapist's own therapy and supervision should be able to offer some help here.

Outmoded treatment?

When Franz Alexander (1950) recommended psychoanalytic psychotherapy for patients with duodenal ulcer it was at a time before the role of helicobacter in gastric ulcer was properly understood. Psychotherapy therefore appeared to offer the best hope of a cure. In some cases it seemed to help. But these days, antibiotics are rightly considered its first and most effective treatment option. Is it possible that the attempt to work psychotherapeutically with trans-people is an equivalent anachronism; a throw-back to an age before effective medical treatment was available? Certainly many people report satisfaction with surgery and hormones. But unlike the treatment for gastric ulcer, serious harm results from the medicalisation of transsexualism. Hormones and surgery cause permanent sterility and damage body integrity and function, without actually changing a person's biological sex at the chromosomal level.

Helicobacter can also be identified under a microscope. But a look at the research (see Withers, 2015; Dreger, 2015) reveals that there is no credible evidence of an equivalent physical factor at work in gender dysphoria- despite widespread misconceptions to the contrary. Since it is not a physically identifiable medical condition, in my opinion gender dysphoria should properly be regarded as 'medically unexplained'. For these reasons it seems to me that surgery and hormones should be a last resort rather than the treatment of choice. It would be possible to argue that such treatment should be banned altogether, like the surgical removal of healthy limbs in people who suffer from 'body identity integrity disorder' (see Muller, 2009). But it is not necessary to accept this argument in order to value thinking about trans-phenomena psychoanalytically.

Some authors still claim there are underlying biological causes for gender dysphoria, despite acknowledging it is not an identifiable medical condition (see e.g. Zhou et al, 1995). They suggest that unusual developments in the foetal brain can predispose a person to discrepancies between their bodily and 'brain' gender and that gender dysphoria can result from this. I am an analyst not a neuroscientist. But basing such claims on six MTF (male to female) cases (as Zhou et al do), all examined on autopsy after a lifetime on female hormones, five of them without testes, strikes me as a statement of faith rather than an evidence-based scientific hypothesis (see e.g. Breedlove, 1996). Meanwhile neuroscientists such as Professor Gina Rippon (2013) assert that there is no evidence that male and female brains are 'hard-wired' differently and hence no biological explanation for gender dysphoria. By contrast there are several plausible accounts of possible psychological factors at work in it. Here are four of them.

1) Sophie and the fear of sexuality

At the age of twelve, Sophie publically identified herself as FTM transgendered. Since coming out, her/his school, friends and family have all been affirmative of her/his new male identity as Robbie. Robbie has been much happier, more confident and is doing better at school than Sophie. For ease of expression I will generally refer to Sophie/Robbie as 'she' prior to coming out and 'he' post coming out. I am aware, however, that this avoids the question of the role of biology in determining gender identity and that from a psychological perspective the sharp divide between before and after coming out could itself express a powerful dissociation between male and female elements in Sophie/Robbie's personality (see section 3).

Sophie had always been a 'masculine' child declaring from an early age that she would be a man when she grew up; apparently without any prompting from her parents. Now aged thirteen, as Robbie, he has begun to be faced with some dilemmas. Should he try to find a way to live with his 'gender dysphoria', by for instance adopting a 'gender fluid' role and refusing to identify exclusively with either pole of the binary male/female dyad, or should s/he perhaps identify as a 'butch' lesbian? Will Robbie be able to find a way of celebrating his sense of being male socially; without the need for any medical intervention? Or would he do better to affirm that male identity by transitioning medically? The latter course would probably involve taking hormones to delay puberty and might lead eventually to testosterone treatment, a double mastectomy and full surgical transition. Of course medical treatment would have serious consequences for his/her future prospects of childbearing, breast feeding, erotic development and sense of identity. Our psycho-social sense of who we are can change over time in a way our biological sex does not.

Robbie is on a waiting list for the Portman Clinic in London. Clients at the clinic can be prescribed puberty-supressing hormones while they consider their best course of action. Should they eventually decide on full transition, they will not then have experienced adulthood in 'the wrong' body. Nor will they have undergone the irreversible changes of puberty. As already mentioned the hope seems to be that they will then be better able to pass as their chosen gender and that this will reduce the alarmingly high post-operative self-harm and suicide rates (Dhejne, 2011). Robbie has shown no signs of feeling suicidal to date. But demands for the Portman Clinic have increased by 1400% over the past six years (Di Ceglie, 2017) and he has now been waiting for over a year. During that time his/her breasts have begun to develop. Robbie's parents, who have been supportive of their child's trans-identity to date, became concerned recently when s/he began talking positively about having them surgically removed.

A little girl's childhood fantasy of growing up to be a man is not uncommon. Several of my patients who are not trans have reported it. But Robbie is not actually one of my patients so I can't claim to fully understand his transgenderism. I see one of his parents. For many years, the couple have been living in a de-eroticised quasi-stability for reasons I am unable to discuss without breaching client confidentiality. From my perspective though, I cannot help wondering whether the advent of Sophie's puberty threatened the family's fragile stability by introducing the dangerous subject of (female) sexuality. Could Sophie have unconsciously sensed anxiety within the family associated with this and come to think of it as a problem in her own body? Perhaps these anxieties triggered the return of her childhood fantasy of being male and identifying as trans appeared to offer a way out of them. If this is the case, then I fear that the medicalisation of Robbie's trans-identification, were it to occur, could amount to the sacrifice of Sophie's breasts at the altar of her parent's inability to tackle their sexual and relationship difficulties.

Robbie's parents continue couple therapy together and spend time with one another and with their children. This is a family that seems willing to try to relate emotionally and think psychologically, despite their difficulties. So it seems entirely possible that Robbie will be able to find a way to celebrate his male identification (should it persist) that does not involve surgery and hormones. If his gender dysphoria does continue to trouble him however, perhaps some good family and/or personal therapy could assist him in this task.

Unfortunately there can be a powerful compulsion to the medical route once it is embarked upon. Well-meaning but uncritical media affirmation and peer and trans-activist 'support' can accelerate its momentum by branding people who question medicalisation transphobic. Surgery and hormones appear to offer a socially-sanctioned way for a family such as this to avoid their psycho-social issues. But, as Ken Zucker rightly pointed out , that route closes down important aspects of the experimentation and search for identity that is normally part of a person's development well into their mid-twenties (Arnett, 2000).

2) The role of mind-body dissociation

Psychoanalytic theory is a difficult subject to write about for an intelligent but non-analytically informed audience. It is all too easy to get drawn into over-simplification on the one hand or over-complication on the other; but I will try.

The term *dissociation* is used in different senses in different analytic schools and its importance is given different weight by them. Historically Freud (see Hacking, 1995) tried to distinguish himself from his contemporary Pierre Janet by using the term as little as possible and largely replaced it with the term *repression*. Analysts such as Jung and Winnicott retained it however, finding a special place for it along-side repression.

Contemporary analysts such as Bateman et al (2010) following Freud (1915b), regard repression as a neurotic defence mechanism which forces unwelcome ideas out of consciousness by means of a 'downward pressure' pushing them into the unconscious. Here the repressed ideas' attempts to return to consciousness are resisted by a censor and they are only able to come back in disguised form. They may do this as a symptom that makes no medical sense, but represents the repressed idea symbolically: - or as a dream, 'Freudian slip' or symptomatic act that does the same thing.

If repression is conceptualised as a *vertical* force within a unified individual like this, then dissociation can be thought of as a similar *horizontal* force (see e.g. Kalsched, 2013). Dissociation pushes incompatible ideas and experiences outside the individual sideways. From this position they are denied the symbolic return to consciousness of repressed ideas. Instead, fractures in the unity of the person are set up without being consciously experienced. In its most extreme form this can manifest itself as dissociative identity disorder (DID) or multiple personality disorder as it used to be called. The Dutch-born American psychiatrist Bessel Van der Kolk (1996) calls this *tertiary dissociation*. He distinguishes it from *primary dissociation* where an unbearably painful reality is treated as if it was a dream and *secondary dissociation* in which the mind becomes dissociated from the body. It is *secondary dissociation* that is relevant in the present context. A transgendered person can be regarded as having identified with the mind of one gender while dissociating from their oppositely gendered body (Withers, 2015).

In moments of trauma, most of us have experienced feeling numb or cut off from our body. Some have even seemed to look on from somewhere outside it. These are both forms of temporary secondary dissociation. They could be understood as normal attempts to protect our subjective sense of self from the fragmentation that might result from being fully emotionally embodied in the presence of the trauma. Instead, such emotions may become isolated in the body and cut-off or encapsulated there in the hope that a time will come when we are able to deal more effectively with them. As the trauma specialist Babette Rothschild (1999) put it; the body remembers.

Dealing with the trauma might be as simple as mother kissing her baby better. Or it might take the more dramatic form of falling shaking and crying into the arms of a loved one to whom we repeatedly relate the traumatic incident until, eventually, we can bear it. At this point we become able to dream, talk, feel and think about the incident without dissociating. The traumatic experience has become integrated into our personal, bodily and narrative history and situated in sequential space and time. Feeling emotionally and physically held can be of central importance for the safe return to embodiment; especially in early life when we are building up the inner resources necessary to deal effectively with life's inevitable later traumas.

If a person is traumatised repeatedly and/or deprived of the inner resources to deal with their traumas by virtue of *insecure attachments*,

(Schore, 2012) such temporary mind-body dissociation can become more permanent. As the psychoanalyst Donald Winnicott (1949) put it, under these circumstances the psyche can become 'seduced' out of its original unity with the body to set up home in a disembodied, devitalised mind. From here the mind/psyche attempts to omnipotently control its internal and external environment; without ever really feeling relaxed or secure. Instead it lives in a state of constant hyper-vigilance. Disembodied emotional numbness may then alternate with occasional terrifying feelings of being emotionally overwhelmed.

Under these circumstances the psyche's return to embodiment becomes extremely problematic. The severity of the repeated traumas makes them far harder to deal with, while the deprivation of inner resources causes the person to fear that a return to the body will lead to breakdown (Winnicott, 1963). Emotion associated with both the repeated traumas and the deprivation, become encapsulated in the body and must be faced if the psyche is to return there. But that way lays madness, or so it seems to the dissociated psyche. More radical measures such as surgery may then appear to be a more viable way of coping.

Chris

Chris had had negative experiences of masculinity from an early age. His father was prone to violent alcohol-fuelled rages in which he threw knives and attacked Chris's mother. He sexually abused Chris's elder brother and left to join the circus when Chris was four. Chris's mother then took up with the milkman. He was a passive man whom she could manage; but she treated him with contempt. She dressed Chris in girl's clothing from an early age and implied through her actions that she could only really love him if he identified as a girl.
From his teens onward Chris enjoyed dressing up in women's clothing, watching himself in the mirror and fantasising about making love with himself. Throughout his twenties and thirties he had heterosexual relationships, at least one of which had a powerful sado-masochistic component. By his thirties he had become convinced he was transsexual and surgically transitioned in the early nineteen eighties. When he woke up from the operation to remove his penis the first thing he said was 'I feel as if all my anger has been cut out'.

When he came to see me for analytical psychotherapy some nine years later, he had decided to try to return to living as a man. He was in a stable, loving relationship with a woman, but still troubled by rages and periodic deep depression. He had come to believe that his identification of himself as a woman had been fuelled by the twin desire to win his mother's love and dissociate himself from his father. He wished he had had analytic therapy prior to surgery, but acknowledged that he might not have been able to use it. A 'supportive' transsexual and medical community had affirmed his hope that surgery would help him feel more at home in his own body. It was only with the benefit of hindsight that he came to see his transition as a socially-sanctioned attempt to evade his complex psychological issues by dissociating from them further. Of course by then it was too late to get his penis back.

From the present perspective, it is the encapsulation of his negative experiences of masculinity in his penis that is of special interest. This part of his body had become the site of overwhelmingly shameful feelings. Those feelings included his own rage and disgust about his sexuality as well as the negative experiences of masculinity internalised from his father and step-father. In addition, his mother's disgust at all things male had deprived him of the inner resources required to process the traumatic feelings imprisoned in his body at precisely the point he most needed them. No wonder surgery had seemed such an attractive option. Of course it hadn't helped. It was what he had dissociated from and attempted to encapsulate there- not his penis itself-that was the problem (see Withers, 2015 for a fuller discussion of this case).

John

When John came to see me some years later, he presented himself as a man who thought of himself as a woman, but wanted therapy before transitioning. So I had high hopes of putting my experience with Chris to good use. It turned out however that John was determined to have surgery. He regarded my attempts to explore any links between his psycho-social-sexual issues and his wish for full transition as at best a failure on my part to understand his identification as trans and at worst an expression of my transphobia. He demanded that I both support his wish for surgery and affirm his condition as normal and healthy. I had trouble accepting this. It seemed to me that John was voicing a logical inconsistency that lies at the heart of a certain strand of contemporary 'trans-affirmative' thinking. That thinking asserts that there is nothing pathological about transgendered states while simultaneously demanding the right of access to hormones and surgery. But if there really is nothing wrong with people who identify as trans, why is such radical medical treatment necessary? On the other hand if there is something wrong then surely it is legitimate to ask what that is and whether there are viable alternatives to medicalisation. John left therapy after two sessions, presumably in the hope of finding a more 'trans-affirmative' therapist.

If Chris's case demonstrates how the denial of psychological factors can lead, via trans-medicalisation, to irreversible physical and severe emotional damage, then John's shows how difficult it can be, in today's 'trans-affirmative' climate, to prevent that damage. Proper analytic work is all too easily dismissed as arising from ignorance and transphobia. What did people who might today identify as trans do in the days before medicalisation and affirmation created this prejudice against working psychotherapeutically?

3) Winnicott's case: The role of male-female dissociation

In February 1966 the psychoanalyst Donald Winnicott read a paper to the British Psychoanalytic Society describing his analysis of a patient who today would very probably have identified himself as trans. Perhaps we could learn something from this work of Winnicott's, which took place at a time before trans-affirmation and medicalisation became so ubiquitous?

In addition to his 1966 paper, Winnicott left some case notes dated 1959 and 1963. From these we gather that his patient was a doctor in his middle age with a family, a series of marriages and girl-friends, potency issues and a history of struggling with, but not acting on, homosexual feelings. We are informed that Winnicott was the man's fourth therapist; that the previous work had lasted a total of twenty five years; but that something had made it impossible for him to finish therapy. Neither Winnicott nor his patient was able to articulate precisely what that something was. But one day Winnicott was struck during a session by the feeling that he was not talking to a man at all- but to a little girl (in Winnicott, 1989 p 170). When he shared this impression, the patient was massively relieved and said 'If I were to tell someone about this girl I would be called mad'. Winnicott continued:

> The matter could have been left there, but I am glad, in view of subsequent events, that I went further. It was my next remark that surprised me, and it clinched the matter. I said: "It was not **you** that told this to anyone; it is **I** who see the girl and hear the girl talking, when actually there is a man on my couch. The mad person is myself.

Before going on to discuss this intervention in more detail, I will pause to ask an obvious question. What makes me think that this patient would have self-identified as trans in today's cultural climate? After all, both Winnicott and his patient were clear that he was in fact a man. Some years earlier Winnicott had already noted (in 1989 p77) his patient's 'far-reaching delusion which he has always had that he is truly female'. The acknowledgement of Winnicott's own madness in the above session enabled him to formulate the following interpretation in the very next one:

> **The girl I was talking to, however, does not want the man released,** and indeed she is not interested in him. What she wants is full acknowledgement of herself and of her rights over your body....The only end to the analysis that this girl can look for is the discovery that you are in fact a girl.

An identification of himself as trans would have confirmed the rights of the girl over his body and medicalisation would have reinforced the dissociation between his male and female sides. But at this stage of his analysis, Winnicott's interpretation enabled his patient to begin to repair the dissociation and this helped release him from his interminable analysis. It also enabled him to make sense of and begin to resolve his potency issues. It seems extremely unlikely that he would have reached this point in his twenty five-year therapeutic Odyssey without transitioning, or at least seriously considering the possibility that he was trans-female, today. It goes without saying that the loss of his penis would have had serious consequences for the recovery of his potency!

From a psychoanalytic perspective, every case is unique. But Winnicott's 1966 paper does focus on one feature that may be of general relevance to transgendered experience: - the almost complete dissociation between male and female elements in his patient's psyche. The male element feared being condemned as mad if it admitted the existence of the female element; while the female element wanted to take over and castrate or kill off the male element.

In order to ameliorate this dissociation, Winnicott had to make the interpretation that it was he, and not his patient, who was mad. As he says, he was *surprised* when he found himself making it. Yet this remark proved transformative. It relieved his patient of the fear that *he* was going mad. Not only was Winnicott alive to his own madness and willing to disclose it to his patient, he was able to trust it meant something within the therapeutic process. It had become part of what Thomas Ogden (1994) calls 'the analytic third'; something co-created from their unconscious interaction. Through it dissociation began to be replaced by *reintegration.*

Naturally Winnicott didn't make his interpretation out of the blue. In his notes four years earlier, for example, talking about his patient's sense of having nothing at the centre he wrote:

> He said he felt tightly wrapped round between the legs and he went on to describe the effect of this on his genitals and his capacity to pee. I had a very great deal of material available which enabled me to make the following interpretation. He was telling me in physical terms how his mother conveyed to him when he was a tiny infant that he was from her point of view a girl and not a boy ... the mother did up his napkin in a way that would be appropriate for a girl baby ... (in Winnicott, 1989 p 51)

It was partly as a result of previous work like this that Winnicott was able to trust that his madness meant something. He came to understand that he was identifying with his patient's 'mad' mother when he saw a little girl on the couch. His patient (p190) had carried the conviction all his life that in order to have a relationship with his mother, he had to be a girl. Naturally this is a very serious thing. In evolutionary terms a baby without its mother is not able to survive. So the girl part of the patient felt she had to kill off the male part in order to go on living and every assertion of male potency felt life-threatening.

Of course Winnicott is not perfect. At times he does come across as mother-blaming and unaware of what a hard time mothers (and fathers) can have raising children in the isolation of modern nuclear or single parent families. They may have never even picked up a baby before facing the huge responsibility of having one of their own. But it seems harsh to blame Winnicott for the fact that our society has organised itself in such a way that childrearing practices make it almost inevitable that in the famous words of Philip Larkin (1971) *'They fuck you up your mum and dad, they may not mean to but they do'*. Evolutionary psychologists (Narvaez, 2017; Newman, 2010) would argue that the communal living of the hunter-gatherer societies within which we evolved do not equip us emotionally for the isolation of modern life, despite our relative material success.

Despite this reservation, I find Winnicott's insights astonishing. The importance of his courageous recognition of what we could call the *countertransference-psychosis* has still not been generally acknowledged. Psychosis is usually thought of as something that happens to the patient, not the analyst. Yet in my own work with John it was precisely my inability to recognise and use a similar psychotic element in my countertransference that disrupted our work together (see Withers, 2015 for a discussion of this). Not being afraid to name his own madness and use it therapeutically was a crucial element in Winnicott's successful analysis of a man who today would probably have identified himself as trans. This must give hope that contemporary therapists could work successfully- even with their clients' most powerful dissociations- if they were able to recognise and use their own 'madness' (counter-transference psychosis) in a similar way. Whether or not sufferers from gender dysphoria would be open to such work, is another matter.

4) The role of identification

The above case illustrates how a person may develop a gender identity at odds with own their physical body. Winnicott's patient only felt capable of having a relationship with his mother if he identified as female. In order to do this he had to dissociate from his male body and identify with his feminised mind. As Winnicott says:

> A mother with a baby is constantly introducing and reintroducing the baby's body and psyche to each other, and it can readily be seen that this easy but important task becomes difficult if the baby has an abnormality that makes the mother feel ashamed, guilty, frightened, excited, hopeless. (Winnicot, 1972 p 271)

In this case the 'abnormality' the mother could not tolerate was her child's male body and so identification with that body became associated with an intolerable sense of emotional abandonment by her. Here then is another way in which unconscious psychological factors can influence a person's 'discovery' that their core sense of gender identity is at odds with that of their body.

There is a further way in which identification can play a formative role in the experience of being trans. The psychoanalyst and founder of the Portman Clinic's gender identity service, Antonio Di Ceglie (2009) describes his work with an eight year old boy 'James' who presented as female following the death of the grandmother who had looked after him from the age of six months. As James began to be able to talk about his grandmother in therapy and mourn her loss, his female identification gradually receded.

To his credit Di Ceglie did talk about this case at the recent transgender and psychoanalysis conference I attended. But he was the only analyst I heard attempt to formulate a link like this between psychoanalysis and a person's identification as transgender. He also mentioned (twice) however, that the funding of the Portman Clinic depended upon the Diagnostic and Statistical Manual of the American Psychiatric Association (DSM) continuing to classify gender dysphoria as a mental disorder. This raises worrying questions about who really profits from trans-medicalisation. Is it trans people themselves, or the surgeons, gender identity clinics and drug companies who treat them?

Unfortunately insurance claims and medical grants depend upon clear diagnostic categories and these are reinforced by the myth that biological rather than psychological factors underlie gender dysphoria. The failure to publically challenge this myth, although perhaps well-meant, seems to me to amount to bowing to, rather than challenging, the cultural stigmatisation of mental illness. It also serves to reinforce belief in the appropriateness of trans-medicalisation, with all its potentially tragic consequences.

Returning now to Di Ceglie's point about identification as a substitute for mourning, this is certainly a process I have seen with some of my own trans-clients. There is no specific case I can talk about at the moment without risking the disruption of their therapy. As a general observation however, it seems plausible to me that the recent upsurge in FTM trans-adolescents could be due in part to this phenomenon. Men have become more involved in childcare over the past few decades. But when families break up, it is often still the mother who takes on the bulk of the childcare. Identification with the missing father may then become a way for the daughter to attempt to deal with her resultant pain and anger; especially if she feels the need to protect her mother from the direct emotional expression of her grief. Identifying as male in this way can have the added unconscious consolation of appearing to provide the mother with a substitute for her missing partner.

Conclusion

This chapter has explored some of the ways in which psychoanalysis may be able to offer a viable alternative to trans-medicalisation. Some cases have been discussed in which it seems reasonable to suppose that the fear of sexuality, dissociation between both mind and body and male and female elements in the personality and issues around identification may have been significant factors in gender dysphoria. Some of the therapeutic implications of this have been pointed out.

It has gone on to describe how, from an analytic perspective, a person's traumatic experiences may become encapsulated and lodged within their body via a process of dissociation. Reuniting with that body then feels fraught with the danger of being overwhelmed by the feelings that caused the dissociation to begin with. This can give rise to fear of a kind of 'madness within'. Under these circumstances it is hardly surprising to find that people may attempt to cope by surgically and hormonally altering their body. It must be acknowledged that many people do express satisfaction with such medical treatment. But I would argue that it can reinforce dissociation, making it harder in the long run for people to reintegrate their traumatic experiences.

The chapter went on to describe Donald Winnicott's analytic work with a man who would probably have identified as MTF transsexual in today's cultural climate. On a theoretical level his work draws attention to the possible role of dissociation between male and female elements in the psyche in the transsexual experience. Clinically Winnicott attributed a crucial part of the successful outcome of this analysis to the recognition and therapeutic use of his own madness. We could say that Winnicott's ability to integrate rather than dissociate from 'mad' elements in his own psyche eventually enabled his patient to reintegrate elements in his own psyche that he had previously dissociated from for fear of going mad. The analyst's awareness of his or her own dissociations helps the patient reintegrate theirs.

Even finding a clear physical cause for gender dysphoria would not necessarily imply the need for its medicalisation. Inter-sex people have rightly objected to the pressure to medicalise their condition despite its clear physical features (Dreger 2015). The continued failure to discover such features in gender dysphoria can only add weight to calls to de-medicalise its treatment. If and when de-medicalisation does happen, it seems vital that the suffering associated with gender dysphoria is not dismissed as unreal. The experience of gender conflict between one's mental/emotional and one's physical sense of self can be profoundly disturbing. Finding ways of living with this effectively and creatively is likely to continue to pose a challenge to trans people, therapists and society alike for many years to come.

I would like to thank anyone who has struggled through this chapter while remaining convinced that its arguments perpetuate transphobia. You could be right. I don't think you are, but I am willing to consider that possibility. In return I would like to ask such detractors to consider the following questions. Who is really doing trans-people a disservice? Is it people like me, who try to open up a discussion of possible psychological factors in gender dysphoria, or those who risk shepherding trans-people into mutilating surgery and a lifetime of hormone treatment by closing that discussion down out of fear of stigmatising them further?

References

Alexander F. (1950) *Psychosomatic Medicine,* New York: Norton

Arnett J. (2000) 'Emerging Adulthood: A theory of development from the late teens through the twenties' *American Psychologist:* May 2000

Bailey, J. M., (2003) *The Man Who Would Be Queen: The Science of Gender-Bending and Transsexualism.* Joseph Henry Press

Bateman, A., Brown, D. and Pedder, J. (2010) *Introduction to Psychotherapy: Fourth edition* London and New York: Routledge

Blood and Visions: Reconciling with Being Female (2015) Autotomous Womyn's Press

Boston Process Study Group (2010) *Change in Psychotherapy a Unifying Paradigm* New York: Norton

Breedlove, M. (1996) 'The Chicken-and-Egg Argument as It Applies to the Brains of Transsexuals: Does It Matter?' *Psychologue*, Newsletter of the Psychology Department of the University of California at Berkeley June, 1996

Britton, R. (1989) The missing link: parental sexuality in the Oedipus complex. In R. Britton, M. Feldman and E. O'Shaughnessy (eds) *The Oedipus Complex today: Clinical Implications p.83-103* London: Karnac

Denman, C. (2003) 'Analytic Psychology and Homosexual Orientation' in Withers, R. (ed.) *Controversies in Analytical Psychology* Hove and New York: Routledge

Dhejne, C. et al. (2011). *Long-Term Follow-Up of Transsexual Persons Undergoing Sex Reassignment Surgery: Cohort Study in Sweden.* Open Access

Di Ceglie, D. (2009) 'Between Scylla and Charybdis: exploring atypical gender identity development in children and adolescents' in Ambrosio, G. (ed.) (2009) *Transvestism, Transsexualism in the Psychoanalytic Dimension* London: Karnac

—. (2016) Private conversation following a talk at the Society of Analytical Psychology

—. (2017) Quoting figures from the Portman Clinic website at the conference *Transgender, Gender and Psychoanalysis* The Freud Centre March 11 and 12 2017

Dreger, A. (2015) *Galileo's Middle Finger*: Penguin

Eysenck, H. (1985). *The decline and fall of the Freudian empire* New York: Viking

Foucault, M. (1961) *Folie et Deraison: Histoire de la Folie a L'age classique* Libraire Plon (in French). First published in English in 1967 as *Madness and Civilization* by Tavistock Publications
Freud, S. (1917) *Mourning and Melancholia* Standard Edition Volume XVII London: Hogarth Press
—. (1905) *Three Essays on the Theory of Sexuality* Standard edition Volume VII. London: Hogarth
—. (1915) *Repression* Standard edition Volume XIV London: Hogarth
—. (1916-17) *Introductory Lectures on Psycho-Analysis* Standard edition XV and XVI
Kalsched, D. (2013) *Trauma and the Soul* London and New York: Routledge
Hacking, I (1995) *Rewriting the Soul* Princeton University Press
Jung, C. G. (1951a) *Collected Works* 9.2 Para 20
—. (1951b) See *Collected Works* e.g. 9 part 1 para 82
Larkin, P. (1971) 'This Be the Verse' in Larkin, P. (2001) *Collected Poems* Faber and Faber
Muller, S. (2009) 'Body Identity Integrity Disorder (BIID) Is the amputation of healthy limbs Ethically Justified? *The American Journal of Bioethics.* Taylor and Francis.
Murad M.H. et al (2010) Hormonal therapy and sex reassignment: a systematic review *Clinical Endocrinology* (Oxford) 2010; 72:214-231
Narvaez, D. (2017) 'Evolution, Childrearing and Compassionate Morality' in Gilbert, P. (Ed.) *Compassion, Conceptualisations, Research and use in Psychotherapy* pp. 76-186
Newman, S. (2010) 'Raising Baby Hunter Gatherer Style' in *Psychology Today* posted on-line Oct 12 2010
Ogden, T. (1994) 'The Analytic Third: Working with Intersubjective Clinical Facts.' *International Journal of Psychoanalysis.* 75:3-19
—. (2001) *Conversations at the Frontiers of Dreaming.* Ch. 6 'Reminding the body' Northvale N.Y. and London; Jason Aronson Inc.
Orbach S. (1978) *Fat is A Feminist Issue.* New York: Berkley Books
Rippon, G. et al (2013) 'Plasticity, plasticity, plasticity ... and the rigid problem of sex. *Trends in Cognitive Sciences.* Vol 17 (11)
Rothschild, B. (1999) *The Body Remembers.* London and New York: Norton
Schore, A. (2012) *The Science and Art of Psychotherapy.* New York: Norton
UKCP (2012) *Press Release.* 13.4.2012.
Van der Kolk, Bessel (1996) *Traumatic Stress; The Effects of Overwhelming Experience on Mind, Body and Society* Guilford Press

Winnicott, D. (1949) 'Mind and its relation to the psyche soma'. In *Through Paediatrics to Psychoanalysis.* London: Karnac
—. (1959) 'Nothing at the Centre' In *Psychoanalytic Explorations.* (1989) London: Karnac
—. (1963) 'A note on a case involving envy' In *Psychoanalytic Explorations.* (1989) London: Karnac
—. (1963?) 'Fear of Breakdown' in *Psychoanalytic Explorations.* (1989) London: Karnac
—. (1960) 'Ego Distortion in Terms of True and False Self' In *The Maturational Processes and the Facilitating Environment.* London: Karnac
—. (1966) 'The split off male and female elements to be found in men and women'. In *Psychoanalytic Explorations.* (1989) London: Karnac
—. (1964) 'Psycho-Somatic illness in its positive and negative aspects'. In *Psychoanalytic Explorations.* Boston: Harvard University Press
—. (1972) 'On the basis for self in body'. In *Psychoanalytic Explorations.* (1989) London: Karnac
Withers, R. (2015) 'The Seventh penis: Towards effective psychoanalytic work with pre-surgical transsexuals *Journal of Analytical Psychology* 60:390-412
Zhou, J.N., Swaab, D.F., Gooren, L.J. & Hofman, M.A. (1995) 'Sex difference in the human brain and its relation to transsexuality'. *Nature* 378, 68-70

Acknowledgements

I would like to thank Pema Sanders and Susan Matthews for their help with previous drafts of this chapter. I would also like to thank those who liked, retweeted and commented positively or negatively on some of my posts on Twitter. You gave me the courage to press on in the face of accusations of trans-phobia, without even realising you were doing so. Last and not least; thank you to my clients for the privilege of working with and learning from you and for allowing me to share with others something of what we have discovered together.

Chapter Eleven

Trans Utopias: Transhumanism, Transfeminism and Manufacturing the Self

Jen Izaakson

> 'What about the reshaping of the human body by modern technology?
> I thought that was your project?
>
> That's just a crude sci-fi concept.
> It kind of floats on the surface and doesn't threaten anybody.'
>
> —David Cronenberg's *Crash* (1996), based on the novel by J. G. Ballard

A decisive surge in the concept of gender identity in recent years has left feminists and others struggling to keep up. Academics, psychologists, medical doctors and the general public have found themselves ill equipped to confront the questions and challenges thrown up by a confident and assertive re-conceptualisation of gender. An identifiably critical strand within the feminist movement is nascent, sometimes visible, but often found to be theoretically lacking in addressing post-structuralist accounts of gender. This chapter is an attempt to set out gender identity's specific locus of emergence inside the University. I will suggest, through the use of some anecdotal references, but mainly a theoretical basis, that Transhumanism and Transfeminism require the same application of scrutiny as any other area of thought that advocates medical intervention as a kind of benign utopianism. This extends to a sceptical analysis applied to the reproduction of gender identity through the media and government, rather than straightforward ideological consumption. Critically, Transfeminism and Transhumanism run the risk of increasing gender normativity and pathologising the gender non-conforming mind and body.

There have been many articles written on social contagion as a contributing factor to the growth in gender identity (Youth Transcritical

Professionals, 2016). A lot has also been written about how the rise of gender identity has mirrored its uptake as a discourse in the mainstream media and how questioning its tenets disrupts the lives of those posing them, such as the cases of Alice Dreger (Muller, 2015) Kenneth Zucker (Singal, 2016) and Rebecca Tuvel (Singal, 2017). For this reason, to add an original component I can perhaps, in the grand style of Transhumanist writing and Queer Theory, offer something anecdotal. My own experience, of being classified as 'trans', was at one of the notable centres responsible for germinating gender identity theory. During my undergraduate degree in the Media & Communications Department at Goldsmiths University, without its oddness striking me at the time, I was repeatedly understood to be transgender. This would at times take the form of curiosity, "are you a boy?" "No, a b.o.i?", "No, I mean are you a boy or a girl?" These are invasive questions that occur regularly to androgynous or ambiguously gendered individuals. Other times it would be mocking comments, "Oh, that ladies' bag really suits you! Don't you think you're crap [at being a trans guy] with that?"

In reply I would convey my ignorance on the topic, by shrugging, eye-rolling or simply stating I wasn't trying to be anything in particular in the least amount of words possible. The message to 'get lost', or illustrating that I was lost in the conversation, uncomprehending of the finite cultural references clothing apparently entails, would usually be understood. This phenomenon has been discussed online as 'gender bullying'. Gender bullying roughly means coercion or policing. When it happens in the service of transgenderism it shows how power can be reorganised under a new set of rules, or terms and how 'scenes' or sub-cultures have the potential to operate as 'terrariums'. Other, smaller worlds with the coercive practices of the 'outside world' transposed towards new goals. Of course, once subversion becomes repetitive, actively commanded, or begins to include a commercial aspect, as with surgical intervention, we see why Judith Butler (2008) two decades ago warned that:

> [j]ust as metaphors lose their metaphoricity as they congeal through time into concepts, so subversive performances always run the risk of becoming deadening clichés through their repetition and, most importantly, through their repetition within commodity culture where "subversion" carries market value.

The curriculum of my department, Media & Communications, would underpin the outside atmosphere of a new radical form of gender conformity policing. Goldsmiths Institute of Management Studies are now doing research into Transgender 'quality of life' (Gendered Intelligence,

2016). Cultivate and incubate something and then perform sociological research on it as if it were naturally occurring. The closely fostered terrarium is treated as if it is the world itself.

The understanding that I encountered of gender non-conformity first and foremost perceived as indicative of a trans identity, as a 'lack', discrepancy between 'internal' self-conception and body, is now more ubiquitous. In 2016, I shared a lift with Polly Carmichael, head of the Tavistock Gender Identity Clinic. Looking at me she asked me, 'are you a service user [of a Gender Identity clinic]?' Short hair and attire from Top Man somehow now indicates not a *comfort* with gender non-conformity, but a necessary discomfort and conflict; dysphoria and a wish to transition. This experience is repeated both in real life and online. It occurs in almost any area where gender identity theory is prevalent or available. That gender identity does not threaten to erase the existence of gender non-conformity is not compatible with my decade-long experience as a gender non-conforming adult. It correlates mainly with similar experiences of being repeatedly told at school I was, 'a boy', this time as an insult. One might be launched as an insult and the other an assumption, but both are underpinned by associations of an essentialist character.

    However, there is a central difference. In the usual case of gender policing the person is objectified by someone else: a young female body scrutinised and coerced into coming into line with the gendered expectations of 'girl' 'woman' and femininity. The affects of gender are awarded to sex. The policing of gender non-conformity by those acting with the assumptions of gender identity theory encourages you to objectify yourself: are the affects of gender awarded to your sex out of sync? Are you a female-bodied individual who fails at femininity? If so, alter your sex or find an identity that clarifies this inconsistency. This lack or deficit needs remedy. Defiance in both cases causes confusion and opposition is found. There is no space for outright rejection of these socially imposed regulatory gender rules. This is partly why the cis/trans binary is so reinforced within gender identity discourse and any non-conformity purportedly housed within the 'trans umbrella' (Scottish Trans, undated). Refusing labels and resisting definition is received as an abrasive rejection of trans subjectivities. The terrarium comes to stand in for the world. Refusing its logic is threatening its fragile walls by exposing it as a tiny world within a world, not the entire world itself.

'Trans'(genderism) as New Queer Identity

I can recall a Professor being sympathetic to me after what I felt was a poor paper presentation. I was told by a friend wholly tied to gender identity theory that, 'he was being nice to you as he probably coded you as queer'. Here 'queer' is being understood as a set of cultural signifiers rather than defying a system of social coercion, or, even as affects allotted into masculinity or femininity that challenge the social order. That the Professor in question was an octogenarian philosopher, who likely had little thorough understanding of all things queer, demonstrates how a universal assumption of a subject's ability to culturally 'code' is a false universal ideal encapsulating a kind of short-sighted crassness. That we read others constantly, unconsciously and consciously has been concretised through queer studies, to a strict set of cultural signifiers. The properties of gender are repeatedly formulated as superficial choices, such as clothes, 'performative' styles, rather than affective states or neurosis. These styles can supposedly embody a 'way of being' that can, with the right selection, be a 'queer' embodiment. This always presumes an internal correlation i.e., a male taking on 'women's' attire is necessarily representing a rejection of masculinity. Masculinity here is no longer about social dominance, or entitlement, but dress code. But how people perceive each other is central to affect-theory and goes beyond the bounds of performance. Whereas within the new queer politics picking the right attire, that represents a supposed rejection of gender normativity, is simultaneously thought to demonstrate subscription to queer ideals. 'Queer' in the sense referenced here has in a similar way to gender identity, come to represent a body knowledge or a particular set of ideas (queer theory, whether understood or not), more than dis-uniformity or that which resists definition i.e., its original or proclaimed qualifiers.

As a method of reading or de-coding cultural forms, queer theory is undeniably useful. Within academia, queer theory is applied to art or other cultural objects, like television, cinema etc. The reoccurring facet of queer theory is ever present in that no limitation on its efficacy is set. 'Queer' as a form of critique therefore easily became the identity of someone who could perform that critique, had heard of it, or wanted some association with the ideas that prescriptive, stable subjectivities were flawed conceptions. Queer as an identity does not widely feature within queer theory, but has now for over a decade been an identity for someone, whether they are LGBT or not, concerned with expressing a particular kind of selfhood.

What was once an anti-heteronormative, problematising cultural critique of objects has been transferred to the realm of human subjectivity. As represented in de Bravo's article 'Transutopia', (de Bravo, 2015) which I will discuss below, the object of critique switches from literature to de Bravo's individual experience. This is the trajectory of queer criticism as a whole. The queer spotlight falls not on lived social structures, but cultural productions and the materially de-contextualised individual. Object has been swapped for subject, and subjects are objectified.

As I hope to show the overlapping features of transhumanism, transfeminism, and transutopianism have been forged within the context of the total absorption of a more recent kind of post-Halperin queer theory into academia. The lack of criticism authors and ideas associated with queer theory, and with the wider 'linguistic turn' receive, has allowed queer theory's more abstract, anti-materialist, identity-bound elements to proceed unchecked.

The proposition of medical gender transition is implicitly prefaced with the capacity of technologies to bring about a freeing transformation. The proposed freedom is a bodily freedom, but also, insofar as they can be distinguished from one another, of the mind. A framework of terminology and legislation works in partnership with the medical industry to support and advocate transition as liberation: not just an end to dysphoria through annulling prior physical constraints, but becoming the 'real you' you are 'inside', on the 'outside' (Fahy, 2016).

The utopian aspects orientating the propagation of transition and gender identity are the critical object of this chapter. The 'Transutopia' article is, I will suggest, emblematic of wider trends within transhumanist and 'Queer' writing. Transhumanism, transfeminism and transutopianism will be addressed in turn, but are understood to be overlapping, connecting areas of thought. I will suggest that transfeminism, as the feminist constituent of transhumanism, the idea that humanity can be enhanced via technology, has given rise to the imagined viability of real yet fantastical transutopias; different worlds existing within, but apart from, the world, and not subject to its usual rules and governing. Transutopias have serious implications for our understanding of the future of the relationship between technology and gender, and there are dangers ahead if we uncritically embrace these supposed 'utopias' without also asking if they might not also turn out to be dystopias.

Technology as the Route to Individual Freedom

What does a utopian transhumanism imagine in relation to the body? What is the relationship between the individual body and the utopian image of anther world? Transhumanist thought contains the idea of liberation via bodily augmentation. For example, transhumanist performance artist Stelarc, who implanted a third ear in his forearm (Quinn and Smith, 2015), is described as someone:

> 'whose guiding light is one basic principle: this bag of flesh we walk around in, the human body, is outdated. Obsolete. Past the point of maximum utility. As simple as it is, it's a mind-melting end game to an entire cyborg/transhumanist school of thought' (Motherboard, 2011)

When transhumanism intersects with feminism it becomes 'transfeminism', with the focus on bodily transformation paramount, but with a specifically gendered angle. 2008's *Testo Junk* (Preciado, 2013) perhaps the apex so far in transhumanist/transfeminist literature, is an account by Beatriz, now Paul, Preciado, of a three-month personal experience of taking testosterone. The work is essentially a diary, mingled with theoretical and historical reflections, what Preciado describes as 'autotheory'. Preciado writes 'I don't take testosterone to transform myself into a man, but to betray what society has wanted to make of me ... to feel a form of pleasure that is post-pornographic, to add a molecular prosthesis to my low-tech transgendered identity'. The personal is swapped for the political in a straightforward interchange, with Preciado becoming the empowered actor at the heart of her/his own story. This tendency is repeated throughout the genre. Of course, the political *is* personal and vice versa. It is, or should be, uncontroversial to state how women's bodies in particular have been sites of political intervention, but I will suggest that never before has the body been conceived of as so uniquely individual and so potentially open to modification by hormonal and physical technologies. Here the 'personal' alone has ultimately trumped and displaced the original feminist slogan, detaching itself from the political understood as any kind of collective project.

What does the belief that the individual can become the author of their own body thus entail? The self-declared purpose of transfeminism, as a sub-category of transhumanism, is, according to Preciado, "the displacement of the site of enunciation from a universal "female" subject to a multiplicity of situated subjects. It involves a conceptual overturning of the debates concerning equality/difference, justice/recognition, and essentialism/constructivism in favour of debates concerning the transversal production of differences" (cited in Corsani, 2007). What, though, are the specific implications for this purportedly 'queer intervention' into the female subject? Preciado's logic leads to a potential cancellation of sex as a meaningful category within discourse. Bligh and Bueti (2013) say about the concept of 'transfeminism':

> "Transfeminism is ... concerned with developing a post-binary feminist-political thinking that goes in the direction of undoing the categories of sex and affirming the multiplicity of the subject."

This is a radical divergence from the second wave feminist proposition of the abolition of gender, moving us instead towards a sex abolitionist position.

Transhumanists of all stripes broadly contend that the optimal way towards a better world is through greater use of existing technologies and technological advancement. By incrementally improving human potentialities we will as a species transcend the limitations of our finite, flawed humanity, and become 'post-human'. If this is understood teleologically it is unsurprising that the landscape of the body becomes a centrally contested site and bodily intervention becomes construed as unremittingly desirable, to the point of fetishism.

Where does gender identity come into this theoretical structure? Gender identity is a key driving force behind the escalating demand for more and more bodily technologies. No one at Gender Identity Clinics today is discussing transfeminism, but I suggest that they are making decisions using very similar assumptions. These assumptions are ones that displace the centrality of sex within socialisation, conceiving of the subject instead as a series of decontextualized immaterial multiplicities and differences without a structural relation. More important than ever before is the centrality of 'self-definition' and self-authorship. This is underpinned by the increasingly prominent idea that the self is simply a matter of chosen identification: one's self is whatever you desire it to be. This has not always been the case within the world of bodily transition.

As recently as 2011, psychiatrists at leading Gender Identity Clinics warned against self-declarations. James Barrett (2011: 381) lead clinician at Charing Cross GIC wrote:

> "The least certain diagnosis is that made by the patient, made as it is without any training or objectivity. This uncertainty is not lessened by the patient's frequently high degree of conviction. Neither does the support of others with gender dysphoria help, since conviction leads

people to associate with the like-minded and to discount or fail to seek out disharmonious views."

Only half a decade later during 2016, in direct opposition to this kind of claim, national legislation was proposed to make self-declaration the qualifying pivotal factor of gender identity (House of Commons, 2015).

What is gender identity? Today gender identity theory postulates that all people (even including historical figures for whom the theory would not have applied, such as Joan of Arc) have an internal identity in relation to a body that either does or does not match this identity: gender is thus a universal property of the subject. The varying degree to which this match is absolute, a perfect fit, or whether there is a gap or 'lack' determines how 'trans' (representing the lack) a person is. The very term 'trans' is an abbreviation of the term 'transitioning'/ 'transitioned' (and perhaps also signifies 'transformation' or even a kind of transitory state). Transition is therefore embedded in the very terminology used to signal the so-called mismatch between the sexed body and 'deeply felt internal' gender identity (Yogykarta Principles, undated). So the term gender identity circularly works to identify both 'problem' and solution, creating its own closed loop. As a brief aside, 'Trans' in the contemporary use overwhelmingly refers to transgenderism, not transsexualism (wanting to be the 'other' sex), or transvestisms (cross-sex dressing), and that is the way in which I use it here.

The increasing insistence that bodily intervention is the best (and perhaps only) way to treat gender dysphoria (a felt mismatch between biological sex and gender) appears, on the face of it, to go against medical ethics of non-maleficence. Somehow, for the 'trans' body, its 'wrongness' and 'need' for correction makes any calculated risk on the part of surgeons and psychiatrists worthwhile. At the heart of this new bargaining relationship is a necessary reformation of the body, with gender as an identity-based component that acts as an exception to the applied rules of medical practice.

That it is possible to feel complete, in sync with or achieve a new comfort by obtaining, 'A body that is the real you', is not, though, a completely new utopian ideal. 'Become the real you' (Moran, 2008), 'Be the best you can be' (Neuro Linguistic Programme, undated), 'Show everyone the real you' (Red Dandelion, undated), is recognisable as the carefully crafted self-help rhetoric that is now a billion-pound global industry. Lifestyle regimes are continually repackaged: self-care is presented as a radical reinvention of self-help, food intolerances and 'clean eating' replace diet regimes, all of which are winding their way towards compelling an imagined consumer to change their life by changing themselves. Gender transition, like body commodification more widely, is not methodically new and neither is the central flaw within it: that anyone can achieve unremitting bodily happiness or feeling free in one's own skin is, as anyone who remembers being a teenager can attest, of course pretty much impossible. The contemporary model of aspiration and wellness is not of course constructed by those suffering from dysphoria, but by a rent-seeking constituency of surgeons, researchers and psychiatrists. One only need consider the high-flying (despite its fraudulence) research career of Dr John Money, or the self-professed empire-building surgeon Curtis Crane to witness the rewards (Bloomberg, 2015; Kinsey Institute, undated). The very idea that an earnest class of medical professionals could be working *ethically* to aid treatment of dysphoria under the auspices of our parasitic neo-liberal capitalism requires a special kind of utopian thinking in and of itself. Somehow the endemically coercive nature of the medical sphere is suspended, even for readers of Foucault, when it comes to medical practice in service of gender identity.

To be clear: it is not that measures of happiness or freedom cannot be achieved through sculpting one's body to match a visualised 'ego ideal' or conventional 'ideal type'. Taking sex hormones may well bring satisfaction, but the so-called gate-keepers of medical technologies set no limitation on their capacities to deliver transformational alternation and what it will provide psychologically. De-transitioned woman Carey Callaghan has her own chapter elsewhere in this collection that touches on precisely this matter.

A growing industry has emerged around the supposedly liberatory idea that doctors can design a 'correctly' sexed body, a body of deliverance, accessing a freedom previously withheld (Cassidy, 2016). This approach brings together liposuction, Botox injections, hair transplants, breast augmentation and other procedures. Those who undergo surgery for reasons deemed 'cosmetic' are told of their potential pitfalls and limitations in what is possible. So if someone is fifty years old they are informed they cannot appear nineteen through multiple face-lifts. Gender identity breaks through this usual barrier of cosmetic surgery: the limitations or problems to changing sex entirely are absent from the process and surrounding discourse. That this process is unrestrained in its potential to eradicate all disambiguation between gender identity and body, and that the project is harmless and possible for all, is the utopian core of the idea of transition.

Narcissism in the Absence of Paternality

How did we get here? How transsexualism has come to be replaced by transgenderism is a topic outside the parameters of this chapter, but we can see that there has been a shift in the discourse from desire (the defining feature of transsexualism) to dysphoria and identity (the defining features of transgenderism). The second order of self-narrative has replaced first order representations, such as desires, fantasy etc. This is reflected in how confession forms a supportive arch of trans-utopianism (and therefore also transfeminism). More than in any other genres of writing, particularly those outside of queer theory, isolated anecdotes are used to present potted personal histories that work as indicators of complete pictures. However, this is positive for our purposes in that it allows some insight into the mind of the writer and also how they construct their worlds.

The features of private history or family life could perhaps be understood as narcissism and perhaps nothing more, but today the personal anecdote has become a powerful vehicle for the genre, even appearing, unusually, within peer-reviewed academic journals. Anecdotes can serve as a record of experience, to underscore a point with a real life example, but the testimonial storytelling in contemporary transhumanism has a curious absence of actors. Interactions are typically missing. The script we're most often reading is a one-person monologue. Other characters are structured entirely relationally to the writer. Psychoanalytically this renders them 'self-objects'. Objectification of oneself and others is a reoccurring theme of transhumanism and that of queer theory writers that overlap with its territory, such as Lee Edelman and Jack Halberstam (Halberstam, 1995). Gender identity theory finds fertile ground here. The emphasis on pronouns as a matter of 'literal' violence – of life or death – is the most clear example: thinking of oneself as a 'she' or 'zie' is to grammatically switch from thinking of ourselves as a subject to an object.

de Bravo's paper '*Transutopias*', treated here as an example of the tropes of this kind of writing, switches from a paragraph about the children's classic *The Wizard of Oz*, to literary descriptions of personal events. The core image for De Bravo in the text is that of a terrarium. Again, terrariums are defined as sealed transparent globes or enclosed containers, traditionally to display plants, but sometimes to house small creatures. A world within a world. Likely accidental, this image nevertheless works to demonstrate the specific kind of world transutopianism imagines. The conclusion of de Bravo is this: 'so much of the larger world lay hidden from me and beyond my control, while this more perfect one within it, contained in glass, belonged to me alone'.

There is possessiveness not just in this single statement, but throughout, "in the forest green bedroom that once belonged to my mother, I ruled over twigs" (de Bravo, 2015). Only in reference to fiction, *The Wizard of Oz*, does de Bravo use pronouns such as 'she' or 'he' consistently to refer to characters. In de Bravo's real life all the characters are "my grandmother", "my bedroom" (even in someone else's house), "my car", "my single mother". The possessive is used in such a way that omits relation to time or relational structure. A childhood bedroom is not, 'my childhood bedroom in my mother's house', just "my room" (in whose home? The grandparents or the single mother's? We are not told.)

That the film *The Exorcist* was reportedly filmed, 'in [de Bravo's] neighbourhood' making it apparently doubly terrifying. It could reveal the movie's scripted nature, rendering it harmless film reel. But not, as here, outside events in the world derive meaning only in relation to ourselves. It is not controversial to notice this as the classic formulation of narcissism. De Bravo writes, "It was liberating to believe in these parallel universes", and I can certainly imagine how. It is only in works of fictions that any other forms of experience other than de Bravo's exist. The characters of *The Wizard of Oz* are rife with their own perspectives, albeit according to de Bravo's reading. But in de Bravo's own world, as described, it is a stand-in for the world itself. In her series of heavily personal anecdotes the actors act only in relation to de Bravo. There is no other narrative bar the author's. This is an inevitability of the possessive grammatical method described before. It also serves a psychic purpose. Psychoanalysis refers to this tendency as rendering 'objects as facts'. Fact is a disputable category but, what 'objects as facts' refers to, is the swapping of our own internal experience for external reality. If I dislike the weather today, the weather was bad. If I am afraid, the thing I am afraid of is frightening. The characterization of the external object is defined by an internal state.

There is a lack of external structuring qualities. Temporal structures are absent. A year is mentioned at one point and an age at another, but these situate the writer's life events with no particular bearing. No connection to the timing of events is made creating a sense of negative structure-less-ness or timelessness. It is the author who is not just centred, but the sole constant quantity. This would leave the author defining all relations, as indeed de Bravo attempts, but its impossibility simply accentuates the absence of relationality. A negative structure that features only in relation to the subject contains only those representations (thoughts, feelings, fantasies) that are self-representations. Self-representation as the only available way of experiencing creates a structure similar to a hall of mirrors. Objects (other people) to the subject (ourselves) are merely self-objects. Others are perceived as parts of the self, as a way to avoid separateness. This is the classic encasing reality narcissists face. This is not to call de Bravo a narcissist, but to illustrate the psychic arrangement we are invited into by this style of writing and thinking. Why is this so important? To understand how it is that trans-utopianism, like its cousin trans-feminism, is characterized by an image of selfhood in exclusion to all else.

A lack of relationally and temporality within psychoanalytic discourse, both Freudian and Lacanian, is immediately recognizable as lacking in paternal functionality. The paternal, most commonly associated within patriarchy as the father, though it can any other third entity, be it a person of any sex or external force that facilities a third between mother and child. Being with the mother (the representative of the maternal function - original object or, in common parlance, the main carer) exclusively is not possible i.e., other people also exist. The paternal function introduces the realization that the mother leaves and returns of her own volition; that the mother has desires of her own; that there is a world beyond the mother/baby dualism for the infant to navigate; that hierarchies exist.

The third paternality is responsible for facilitating a structuring relation to time, comprehending limits or negation. The process of structuring takes place through prohibition, i.e., we come to understand we cannot be seven years old forever. The most common example is a child hearing 'no' leading to the recognition that whilst the world is full of possibilities, it also contains impossibilities. This vital function also makes the child realize that there is not only themselves and the mother. The mother at first represents oneness and the entire world of the early infant. Paternality is how we recognize there is a world beyond our own experience that involves boundaries, consequences and other separate beings. A third paternality also demonstrates generational gaps; not only representing a prohibition to incest, but a structure of relations that includes temporal distinctions.

All these vicissitudes of the paternal combine towards maturational separation, introduce time to the mind of the subject, facilitate the inauguration of systems of shared meaning (such as language), establish a tolerance for shades of grey beyond yes and no, etc. So, the paternal necessarily includes consequences, bestows rules, limits and other vital components to structure the mind through negation. The paternal is the negative domain of what is 'not'. When this installation fails it gives rise to psychosis. The mind develops what Lacanians refer to as a 'psychotic structure' (Vanheule, 2011). Psychosis is experienced as timeless because it represents a lack of temporal structure.

Paternal authority is, I suggest, absent in transutopianism. Its absence is in fact explicitly celebrated, as if railing against hierarchy is the same as failing to recognize its presence. I would go so far as to say a major characteristic of trans-utopianism is that the absence of 'the law' and defines its thought. De Bravo (2015) writes:

> "My utopia would be a land of unregulated joy and extreme but always surmountable danger. Arriving there could never be as easy as pushing past coat sleeves smelling of naphthalene. It would involve relinquishing control, but not to parents, teachers, or anyone in authority."

Where can the beginning of this tendency of not delineating limitations or impossibilities be traced to in regard to gender? In queer theory the lack of boundary is similar. In queer theory, gender is conceived as discursive. Almost any contemporary scholar working within the Humanities would agree that is a correct assessment. What is never part of the discussion is that gender is not 'limitlessly' discursive. Gendered subjectivities are highly constituted therefore they are necessarily constrained within a temporality. But constraint, incapacity, limitations are somehow not included in the constitution of subjectivity when viewed through the queer lens. Structural subject positions are, by their being as positions within a structure, curtailed in malleability or manoeuvre. But if gender or sex or identities no longer require any relation to a structure, then the individuals defining themselves in this way have a 'utopian' total freedom so to do.

The potentiality of subjectivity defines itself, not the structure it takes place within or any relation to it. If a subjectivity is available, it can seemingly be garnered. Identities come to be adornments. Consumed or disposed of without ever relying on any material relation. But this is a false potential, as whether a subject recognizes 'the law' or not, all sociality takes place within a horizon far beyond the subject as an individual. The subject negotiates at all times this structure and is structured by it, with very little ability to influence the structure itself. There is also the small matter of power; who gets to define into a certain group cannot escape power. A black person is far less likely to be accepted as a transracial white person, than a white person orchestrating an entry into blackness. This is demonstrably verifiable by the legitimacy white supremacy still enjoys and the lack of recognition of cultural appropriation of blackness by white entertainers, amongst many other examples.

However, smaller worlds can be more readily structured. Transutopias differ from theoretical transhumanism in that spaces have been constructed not of a future wider world, but a minor world that pretends the rest of world exists as it does. Surgeons promise individuals that they can transform their bodies in a way technology often cannot deliver. The inability to 'pass' and how that will feel at the end of a series of medical interventions is not a regular part of Gender Identity Clinic assessments. Sex transition is discussed in classrooms or Internet forums as if it is entirely possible for dimorphic species like humans to actually change sex. This is how one cultivates a terrarium. Language is no longer a shared system of meaning, but one's own personal set of signifiers, though everyone else is not just invited, but commanded, not to share in, but submit to.

There is one inevitable conclusion to this. Lewis Carroll, for one, understood the inherent power of words in deciding meaning and how this is a way to power, as this prescient passage in *Through the Looking Glass* reflects:

> 'I don't know what you mean by "glory"' Alice said.
> Humpty Dumpty smiled contemptuously. 'Of course you don't — till I tell you. I meant "there's a nice knock-down argument for you!"'
> 'But "glory" doesn't mean "a nice knock-down argument"' Alice objected.
> 'When I use a word' Humpty Dumpty said, in rather a scornful tone, 'it means just what I choose it to mean — neither more nor less.'
> 'The question is' said Alice, 'whether you can make words mean so many different things.'
> 'The question is' said Humpty Dumpty, 'which is to be master — that's all."

Ruse of the Naturally Occurring Phenomenon

For the transhumanist quality of gender identity to remain then its supposedly universal and trans-historical nature must be reinforced wherever possible. This is seen in the historical posthumously 'transing' of gender non-conforming figures such as Hans Christian Anderson, Kurt Cobain and Joan of Arc. This conceptualization of transgenderism differs strikingly from social constructionism, regularly typified as a 'reveal' or what has been operating behind or underneath socially performed gender. An authentic true self. One reason that desistance and de-transitioned individuals are such a threat to gender identity ideology is because they show that gender is not essential or absolute. Ambiguity and doubt have no place within the strictures of gender identity and are threats the market models of the growing vocation of private 'gender identity specialists'.

Gender identity has a circular role in accelerating technologies, both producing the need for and continually reinforcing their necessity through consumption. This cycle can be observed if gender identity is detected as not naturally occurring, so the industry and rent-seeking class of clinicians who rely on it are invested in its appearance of naturalness.

Parents are encouraged to consider children who defy gender stereotypical behaviour as showing signs of being a Trans infant. Gender non-conforming individuals are second-guessed as 'Trans', despite their protestations. The sum of these conclusions founds the idea that there is a consistent, pre-existing category of subjects only now receiving recognition. A trans-historical, hidden demographic, with its own unique ontological reality, is finally coming into view. The naturalness of this category is what the persistent theme of 'trans' as a new civil rights frontier relies on. The 'rights' mentioned here are framed exclusively in relation to the transgender conceptualisation, as opposed to transsexual or transvestite identities, the latter two having been fully subsumed into the former.

I conclude with the problem that is perhaps the most urgent, the question of what the term gender actually means. Whether gender means a system of socially imposed norms, refers to masculine or feminine components of psychic life, or as gender identity theory extols, signifies innate essences, is the battleground over which both women's rights and gender identity in the future will live or die.

References

Barrett, J. (2011) *Advances in Psychiatric Treatment,* Vol. 17 *doi: 10.1192/apt.bp.109.007484*

Bligh, R. and Bueti, F. (2013) Editorial, *Journalment,* 2013

Bloomberg (2013) *Meet The Surgeon Sought After By Transgender Men* October 26th 2015, https://www.bloomberg.com/news/articles/2015-10-26/meet-the-surgeon-sought-after-by-transgender-patients

Butler, J. (2008) Preface, *Gender Trouble: Feminism and the Subversion of Identity*, London: Routledge

Cassidy, S. (2016) *Gender identity issues among children increase tenfold in six years: Latest Gender Identity Development Service figures show children as young as three being referred to the NHS*, The Independent, February 11th 2016, http://www.independent.co.uk/life-style/health-and-families/health-news/gender-identity-issues-among-children-increase-tenfold-in-six-years-a6868306.html

Corsani, A. (2007) *Beyond the Myth of Woman: The Becoming-Transfeminist of (Post-) Marxism,* Substance, Vol. 6, No. 112

de Bravo, B.F. (2015) *Transutopia,* Fourth Genre: Explorations in Nonfiction, Vol. 17, No. 2 (Fall 2015), 73-84

Edelman. Lee, (2004) *No Future: Queer Theory and the Death Drive,* Durham, North Carolina: Duke University Press

Fahy, J. (2016) *Swapping Sex to be the Real 'You',* http://www.swissinfo.ch/eng/society/transgender_swapping-sex-to-be-the-real--you-/42234396, Swiss Info, June 28th 2016

Gendered Intelligence (2016) *Quality of Life Survey,* http://genderedintelligence.co.uk/quality-of-life-survey October 2016

Halberstam J. and Livingston, I. (1995) *Posthuman Bodies,* Bloomington: Indiana University Press

House of Commons (2015) *Transgender Equality: First Report of Session 2015 -16,* House of Commons Women & Equalities Committee, December 8th 2015

Kinsey Institute (undated) *About Dr John Money,* https://kinseyinstitute.org/about/profiles/john-money.php

Moran, S. (2008) *The Real You, Experience Life.* https://experiencelife.com/article/the-real-you

Motherboard (2011) *Stelarc, The Transhumanist Artist With Three Ears,* http://motherboard.vice.com/read/from-the-motherboard-vault-stelarc-- 2 September 29th 2011

Muller, Martin N (2015) *Review of Alice Dreger's Galileo's Middle Finger: Heretics, Activists and the Search for Justice in Science,* New York: Penguin Press

Neuro Linguistic Programme (undated) *Be The Best You Can Be,* NLP Practitioner, http://nlppractitioner.uk.com/945

Preciado, Paul B. as quoted in Corsani, p135, Corsani. A, 106 – 138, *Beyond the Myth of Woman: The Becoming-Transfeminist of (Post-) Marxism,* Substance, Vol. 6, No. 112 (2007)

Preciado, P. B. (2013) *Testo Junkie: Sex, Drugs and Biopolitics in the Pharmacopornographic Era,* New York: The Feminist Press

—. (2008) *Pharmaco-Pornographic Politics: Towards a New Gender Ecology* Parallax, Vol. 14, No. 1, 113

Quinn, L. and Smith, L. (2015) *'I've got something up my sleeve': Nutty professor with Australia's creepiest laugh shows off the ear he grew on his ARM using stem cells in bizarre TV interview,* http://www.dailymail.co.uk/news/article-3194396/He-s-got-sleeve-Australia-s-nutty-professor-Stelarc-shows-surgically-grown-ear-bizarre-TV-interview.html Daily Mail Online, August 12th 2015

Red Dandelion (undated) *Reveal the Real You!*
http://www.reddandelion.co.uk/life-coaching-tips/reveal-the-real-you

Scottish Trans (undated) *Transgender Umbrella,*
http://www.scottishtrans.org/trans-rights/an-intro-to-trans-terms/transgender-umbrella

Singal, J (2016) *Fight Over Trans Kids Got a Researcher Fired,* http://nymag.com/scienceofus/2016/02/fight-over-trans-kids-got-a-researcher-fired.html, New York Magazine February 7th 2016

—. (2017) *This Is What A Modern-Day Witch Hunt Looks Like,* http://nymag.com/daily/intelligencer/2017/05/transracialism-article-controversy.html New York Magazine May 2[nd,] 2017

Vanheule, S. (2011) *The Subject of Psychosis: A Lacanian Perspective.* Hampshire: Palgrave Macmillan

Yogykarta Principles (undated) *Preamble* http://www.yogyakartaprinciples.org/preambule

Youth Transcritical Professionals (2016) *Social Contagion,* https://youthtranscriticalprofessionals.org/tag/social-contagion/, November 8[th,] 2016

CHAPTER TWELVE

STANDING UP FOR GIRLS AND BOYS

MICHELE MOORE

The proposal that transgender people and disabled people share the same conditions of oppression is achieving a level of liberal consensus within discussions on the identity struggles of disabled people and those who identify as transgender. Scholars argue a medical authority is applied to understanding transgender people and disabled people that pathologises their bodies and leads to a neglect of the social determinants of difficulty, inequality and exclusion (Stryker and Aizura, 2013). A social constructionist approach to the way in which medical authority guides and shapes the lives of disabled and transgender people reveals it as a reductive theoretical lens through which individuals and groups are regulated. Arguably transgender people and disabled people can forge alliances to empower themselves with alternative identity constructions that reject the way in which dominant medical discourses regulate their lives. The viability of this proposed alliance is powerful because transgender people and disabled people have group identities negotiated in response to social injustice. It is asserted that resistance to the medical model of understanding experience will forge alternative identity constructions for transgender people that will enable resistance of barriers to well-being and inclusion and mobilise collective action to combat injustice and social control. As a scholar of Disability Studies who uses social constructionism as a methodology for understanding the experience of disability and transgender, I arrive at very different conclusions to those outlined above.

In this chapter I argue that alliances should not be made between the disabled people's movement and the transgender movement for the following reasons. Firstly, to reject the medical model for disabled children on the grounds it is oppressive logically requires rejection of the medical model for their gender nonconforming peers. The transgendering of children does *not,* however, escape from the medical model but endorses it. Secondly, ideas from earlier discussions in the history of

Disability Studies provide possibilities for freedom from medicalization for disabled children and offer alternative ways to respond to, and care for the welfare of, children who question gender. Thirdly, the idea that political resistance should take identical forms between transgender people and disabled people is an overly simplistic way of challenging the minutiae of oppression and the social barriers that lead to different forms of exclusion. I argue that transgender activism, unlike disability activism, far from disrupting oppression and promoting inclusion, intensifies surveillance, creates pathology and tightens public control with the effect of manufacturing oppression and exclusion.

I conclude that the proposition that disability and transgender can be politically and theoretically aligned is not progressive, has confusions embedded within it which do not best serve the interests of transgender children and that the struggles of disabled children and their families are undermined if their interests are subordinated to the politics of transactivism. My research into the experiences of parents with children identifying as transgender, and with children themselves, grounds this conclusion.

The medical model and transgender children

I argue that transgender doctrine advocating the transitioning of children does *not* escape from the medical model but actually insists on it. In the UK, as in a number of other countries, pressure on parents to accept medical practices which intervene to transform the bodies of their gender nonconforming children is increasing. Even though there is no evidence base for medical transition of children, parents who worry about medicalization are assured by a number of sources (media, doctors, teachers, transgender activists) that subjecting their child to social and physical gender correction will empower their child, make them less anxious about their personal choices, allow them to 'fit in' socially when they are older and, by implication, facilitate them to have comfortable sexual partnerships as adolescents and adults. This advice is predominant in psychological and National Health Service literature as Brunskell-Evans in Chapter 3 and Davies-Arai in Chapter 2 of this volume have shown. It is advice which negates over thirty years of campaigning by disabled people for understanding that children with impairments are not disabled by their bodies but by the disabling barriers they face in society' (Oliver, 2013).

At the same time, children are being taught that expressing confusion about their gender unquestionably confirms they *are* transgender, that medical reassignment of their body will resolve gender discomfort and that without social and physical intervention they will be likely to self-harm and probably commit suicide. We have seen in various chapters that parents are told if they object to reassignment of their child's body, or even question such procedures, this is indicative of intolerance and transphobia likely to aggravate their child's need to self-harm and almost certainly to lead them to commit suicide. There is a circularity to the logic of transgender doctrine which makes inescapable the view that transgenderism is a self-fulfilling prophecy: children self-identify as transgender, social and medical intervention takes place thus confirming and intensifying the child's self-diagnosis; parents, teachers, other professionals and caregivers are induced to understand gender nonconformity as evidence of transgenderism, to accept transgender doctrine as 'truth' and to collude with social and medical intervention.

The growing number of children identifying as transgender occurs against a backdrop of the media, the internet, medicine, education, social policy and politics, including transactivism. These interconnected influences provide the background to children's everyday lives and currently combine to popularise, and make gender transitioning socially acceptable. This backdrop constructs for children an obvious and definitive set of 'truths' about transgenderism and about their own self-identification as transgender and is normalising gender dysphoria. Children and young people with mental health issues such as anxiety or depression, living with trauma or diagnosed with autistic spectrum disorders are overrepresented amongst children who self-diagnose as transgender but minimal attention is paid to the question of whether and how children's interests are being destabilised by the agenda of transactivists.

What follows is an attempt to illustrate how transgender activism gains traction through sharing some of the empirical data I am gathering with children and families. The story of 'Robert and Her Mother' is an anonymised, typical account from a worried mother and trans identifying daughter taken from their exchanges during the period between 2014 and 2017, based on the mother's subsequent relating of these events to me. This story is offered as a starting point for reflection on contemporary constructions of 'the transgender child' enabling observation of how transgender activism operates, oppresses children and drives exclusion, before moving on to an analysis of what can be learned from trends that have previously been predicated upon children's bodies, making similar promises to children with impairments that their bodies could be reconciled to better fit social expectations.

A Story of Robert and her Mother

'It was a completely out of the blue announcement' her mother said. 'Just after her fourteenth birthday she told me she was really a boy and was going to transition. I was shocked. I told her we had better find out more about it as I never had any idea she thought she was really a boy'. 'I know all about it' said the girl. 'I read everything about it on Tumblr and watched loads of YouTube videos. Just write to my school and tell them I'm going back as a boy in September. I've already told my friends. They call me Robert now and use 'he' pronouns'.

'We had better find out more about it' her mother said again, 'as you never previously showed any sign you felt like a boy. And what do you mean? What do you mean when you say you think you are a boy?' 'I don't really know' said the girl, 'I haven't been a boy yet. Anyway I'm getting testosterone when I'm sixteen and having my breasts cut off. I'm not having bottom surgery'. 'Well then you won't be a girl or a boy will you?' asked the confused mother. 'Have you thought very much about what your life would be like?'

'I knew you would be like this' said the girl. 'On Tumblr trans phobic parents like you who wouldn't accept it made their daughter Leelah throw herself under a tractor. Anyway I can do it even if you don't tell school I can. School have to let me be a boy. They're already letting Emily be William even though his mum and dad said they won't go along with it. William's getting T on his 16th birthday. William says if I live as a boy for two years I can get a letter from Dr Seabrook for the Gender Clinic and do what I want. I know what to say. You just have to say 'I've always known I was a boy' and then they have to let you have T. If anyone tries to stop me I'm just going to say I might have to kill myself. No one can stop me. Everyone knows what you have to say'. 'Do you have thoughts about killing yourself?' asked her mother who was very frightened by now. 'No of course I don't. I'm not a complete idiot mother. I just know what to say. But you had better get used to the idea of having a dead daughter because I am going to be your son'. 'I thought you were a lesbian' her mother said. To which the girl replied 'it's easier to be straight guy than a gay girl.' 'It's true she endured a lot of verbal abuse after she came out as being gay' her mother told me. 'One day she came come home with a bruise on her cheek as a result of being pushed into a wall on the corridor by three homophobic boys. When it happened again school said they couldn't do *anything to help her because the incidents were never in sight of the corridor CCTV'.*

The mother described how:

'... eighteen months later my daughter had spent nearly two years dressing as a boy, binding her breasts for long hours every day. Sometimes two binders layered, hardly able to walk and breathe so having to give up sports. She had her hair cut short at the barber shop, put a badge on her backpack with the trans symbol and wore t-shirts with logos for trans boys. By now she was being treated as a boy by her peers (who never forgot to use the male pronouns). She spent hours online following posture change training for transmen or practicing 'Female to Male Voice training for teenagers waiting to get Testosterone' on the internet. She was endlessly quoting transactivist on-line coaches who urge trans identifying children to get away from their families as fast as they can – one of her favourite quotes for example,

> 'I want you to know' says transwoman Rachel McKinnon PhD in Philosophy. Assist. Prof at College of Charleston 'that it's ok to walk away from unsupportive or disrespectful or even abusive parents. And I want to give you hope that you can find what we call your glitter family. Your queer family. We are out there' (4thwavenow 2017)

By now school work she used to do well was long forgotten. She hardly went out. She was morose, cutting her arms and thighs at night with carbon steel razor blades and saying soon she might get suicidal if she had to wait much longer for testosterone therapy. She was so concerned about her voice not passing as male that she barely spoke. She communicated mainly via email and WhatsApp even if we were in the same room. One day she wrote asking me 'how am I meant to understand the difference between gender confusion and trans? Explain the difference! How else am I going to understand it?' And then a volley of confusion, 'I know trans people say they're born in the wrong body and really they're a boy, I don't understand that because clearly I'm not a boy but I need to be one because it will make me more happy, and when I have more of a male body then I will feel like I actually am one. If someone asks I will say I'm definitely trans because it's the easiest way to get turned into a boy. I'm going to do it anyway so there's no point talking about the dangers any more, I know what they are and I'm still going to do it. I know what to say'.

'I can see you really are unhappy' said her mum *'but I can't support your idea that the reason is because you are a boy trapped in a girls' body'.*

By now the girl easily met the criteria to be diagnosed with Gender Dysphoria in the UK having exhibited 'a strong and persistent cross-gender identification for at least a 6-month duration' (Bressert, 2017). Knowing this, her mother made every excuse she could think of for not talking to teachers or getting a doctor's appointment because she wanted to avoid uncritical affirmation of her child's self-diagnosis feeling sure the child was in a complicated phase of teenage identity exploration but not actually 'a boy in a girl's body'. Terrified of her daughter's escalating withdrawal and self-harm, she nonetheless persisted with the line that they needed to find out more about how girls are turned in to men before they took things much further. Then without any evident sign of change,

Suddenly, another six months on, she emailed again out of the blue, saying 'why did anyone tell me I could be a boy ffs when I can't? Why do people lie? Transgender is a great big lie. I've told my friends not to trans me anymore because it's just stupid. They can call me my real name again because 'Robert' just sounds stupid. I don't know why so many people say a girl can be a boy when obviously they can't.'

To the mother's astonishment, after years of debilitating anguish and unmitigated gender dysphoria, her daughter quietly went back to being a happy lesbian, preferring to wear her brother's cast-offs than fuss with fashion but no longer trying to look or behave as a stereotypical boy. After three years of adamantly identifying as transgender she gradually rediscovered her voice, her laugh, her natural way of walking, picked up her school work, set about growing her hair and applying for university and these days wants never to think about what she calls 'the transgender lie' again.

'Three years thinking she was a boy' said her mother. *'Thank god school didn't get properly hold of it and I managed not to let her anywhere near a doctor. These are sorry times when parents have to hope a distressed and self-harming child won't say a word to adults who are supposed to help them because all of those adults can only celebrate and reinforce the child's confusion. We had nowhere to turn that would have given her options'.*

Transgender activism as oppression

Research demonstrates that more and more parents report their trans-identifying teenagers eventually desist from adopting a transgender identity (Maynard, 2016). This is made much more difficult once social and medical intervention has begun and the child will have to backtrack. Some transactivists argue that children and young people who change their minds about being trans *'were never really trans'* (Herzog, 2017). The problem with this argument, amongst other things, is that current policy and medical practice is to treat all children and young people as *definitely trans* if they have claimed that they are trans for longer than six months. If at some point the girl in the story above had sought support from her teachers or health professional her transgender identity would have been affirmed, leading to social reinforcement of gender confusion and proposals of medical intervention. Transgender activism has a vested interest in making it difficult for trans identifying children and young people to change their minds in order to protect its claims of gender as a biological phenomenon.

The shift from social transitioning to medical intervention is fuelled for adolescents, as trans identity is zealously reinforced over the internet. Typically, trans identifying children dedicate huge amounts of time to 'passing' as the 'opposite gender'. This is time spent anxiously obsessing over how to comply with gender stereotypes. An extract which follows from an online conversation between two young people illustrates the level of dedication that needs to be paid to this. In the following conversation advice is given by a boy, who says he had previously lived as a girl, to a natal girl who says she is really a boy but needs tips on how to perform 'masculinity':

> FtoM: "OK so behaving male seems to be an issue for me. I know I FEEL male inside, but sometimes I act way to girly and I need to work on that"
>
> How to walk like a guy 101:
> When you look at other people make sure you're only looking at either a woman's tits or her ba-donka-donk if she has one.
> Say hi, or mumble something, then quickly walk by.
> Take long strides.
> Clomp a little with all of your foot, and by all means never walk just on your toes or ball of your foot.
> Skip stairs when you're going up, taking two or three at a time.
> Wear larger shoes than you really need.
> Wear larger pants than you really need. (GenderTrender, 2011)

Clearly the performance requirements transgender children seek to induct themselves in to cannot be said to nurture an 'authentic self' or 'gender freedom'. In the pursuit of supposed gender liberation children are made acutely aware of gender related determinants of exclusion and given no option but to cultivate these. The child receiving intensive advice on gender performance says elsewhere that her parents are 'on board with me starting T' demonstrating that social transition goes hand in hand with medical intervention; intervention begets intervention. Hormone therapy also, of course, brokers further confusion since it comprises intervention at the site of 'sex' not 'gender'. First the child misses out on puberty, next an already confused girl has a vagina and a beard, a confused boy has a penis and breast growth. The only way forward for the child is to plough on seeking more and more treatments allegedly to relieve gender dysphoria. As Callahan has explained in Chapter Eight however, gender dysphoria does *not* readily go away with intervention.

Critique of the proposed coalition of disability studies and transgenderism

In watching the fervour to intervene on the bodies of children diagnosed as transgender, I am reminded of a similar eagerness in the 1980s to intervene on the bodies of children with cerebral palsy in order to make them stand up and walk, and thus comply with society's normative standards. Mike Oliver, world leading advocate of disabled people's rights who first examined the social construction of disability and its relationship with society, fought hard against widespread eagerness for correcting the bodies of disabled children through the painful and isolating therapeutic intervention known as Conductive Education. Oliver's resistance was responded to as if he lacked generosity and kindness towards children who had been born to 'suffer' cerebral palsy but allegedly could learn to stand up and walk if only their parents could be persuaded to sufficiently comply with medical regulation of their child's body. Oliver was not shamed in the face of such criticism but redoubled his efforts to speak with fairness and humanity in accordance with principles of the social model of disability, to assert that difficulties of inclusion for any child must not be located within the child and their body but circumvented by paying attention to the removal of material, ideological, political and economic barriers that impose inequality and disability in the lives of children with impairments. Eventually Oliver's refusal to be silenced turned back the tide of medical intervention. He refocussed attention on how discrimination and inequality in an unjust world must be challenged rather than seeking to modify children's bodies in the face of injustice, particularly when it is known proposed intervention will cause harm (Oliver, 1989). Criticism of the transgender trend can be made through the same lens of social constructionism, drawing on the same arguments Oliver made in the 1990s to resist the triumph of the medical model over a social model in the lives of children who are confused about gender.

The medical model of normality permeates transgender doctrine that advises the transitioning of children according to society's normative standards for gender. The idea that the cause of 'misaligned' gender lies in a child's body is central to transgenderism, so that medical intervention can be countenanced even though the inevitable result of such intervention will be a life-long pursuit of difficult and painful physical and psychological transitioning that will uphold and deepen socially constructed gender based oppression and never actually change a person's biological sex. Intervention is made socially acceptable through the key premise that children are born in 'the wrong body': any intervention – medical, educational, psychological, social care and so on – is then deemed to be acceptable as long as enough adults equate a child's wish to be gender nonconforming with the supposedly pathological condition of being 'transgender'. To transpose observances made by Oliver speaking out about harm several decades ago, if disabled children were subject to interventions in school without their parents' permission, taken in to care if their parents should object to intervention, encouraged to reject their own bodies, advised to undergo as yet unregulated hormonal therapies, bind their bodies, plan for experimental surgery, and on top of all this, urged to undertake ableist compliant behaviours 24/7 for the rest of their lives we would regard it not only as unacceptable but as a travesty of the human rights of the child.

Transgenderism as the intensification of control

In contrast to the view of some disability scholars that transgender identity is a form of social transgression and resistance to oppressive cultural norms, I argue that the identification of children as transgender intensifies surveillance, creates pathology and tightens public control. This can be illustrated through the example of education, at the levels of pupil interaction, school policy and their inter-relation.

At the level of pupil interaction, the girl in the story of Robert and her Mother for example, was regulated by numerous sources. Firstly, her peers performed surveillance of her by lauding her as a transboy, an approach they had been instructed to take by a transactivist- led organization brought in to provide an in-schools gender training day. Her friends constantly reminded her of her preferred male personal pronoun if she used the female personal pronoun. Her transgender identifying status immediately conferred popular and exotic status in comparison to her previous lesbian status. She was thus policed to be a transboy, and policed not to be a lesbian. In both instances of policing, the real causality was gender freedom and fluidity. Of course, her peers were in turn regulated to accept transgender doctrine as an explanation for gender variance, not only by the school and special interest groups and activists delivering training, but also by social media, including mainstream broadcast media, which glamorises transitioning and is silent on transcritical perspectives.

Secondly, the girl policed herself, by constant monitoring of her own appearance, behaviour, language and communication frustrated by her awkwardness in performing masculinity and inability to sound like a boy. Performance difficulties were intensified by fear of losing 'face' if her own doubts about her 'boyhood' should begin to surface and so she began to exclude herself from social contact. When she solicited support from transgender adults advising children on the internet, she was routinely told that it is 'normal' for children questioning gender identity to want to self-harm, and that she may feel suicidal if her 'gender variance' was not being unequivocally endorsed. Consequently, when she did start self-harming, she understood this as inevitable and unavoidable. She had no counter-narratives to put a brake on self-harming behaviour. We see from the abstracts above that the girl *talks herself into* acceptance of the suicide trajectory even though she started off thinking she was simply going to manipulate suicide discourse for her own ends.

Thirdly, on the issue of tightening public control, once the transgender identity had been uttered by the girl, the mother, in exercising responsibility for her child had no recourse to public institutions which ordinarily support children and families because they already have in place policies and practices which discourage transcritical conversation. The very institutions set up to facilitate the child's welfare and well-being, had become purveyors of a mono-logical lens through which the child's gender disquiet must be understood.

At the larger level, organizations interested in promoting transgender doctrine to children, have unparalleled access to schools to draw children into conversations concerning their gender and sexual identity. The leading UK Teachers Union, for example, has adopted pro-trans policies giving a transactivist agency (GIRES) permission to supply schools with cartoon books aimed at identifying transgender three to six year olds by asking children if they are really a 'Blur' who belongs in Penguin Land rather than a boy or a girl who belongs in their own world (4thwaveNow, 2015). Little children are taught that if they do not conform to their assigned gender in schools, they can choose a new identity with which everyone, including their own parents, will have to comply. Policies are in place to prevent teachers from asking questions about what they are required to teach. From my own observations I cannot help but be concerned that *'silenced as they are [teachers] are the world's biggest distributors of trans'* (YouthTransCriticalProfessionals, 2016).

By 2015 a peripatetic colleague working in schools across the north of England found she was coming into contact with children and young people identifying as transgender, and transactivists training in schools, on an almost daily basis. She described most teaching staff, allied professionals and parents as operating 'in a grey soup of unfamiliarity, devoid of dialogue' around transgender issues. No questions or discussions were going on in schools about why Trans Training was regularly taking place, about what had been learned, opinions, value of the input – no discussion she noticed, is permitted (Awakening Clinician 2016). It is unclear why or how transactivists have gained unrestrained access to schools when their central messages subordinate children's own ideas about gender to prevailing politics of vested interest groups. Reflection on parallels between the transgender movement and the disabled people's movement reminds me that disabled people's organisations have not ever had similar admittance to freely share their struggles, agency and perspectives with children and young people. At the moment children and young people are being influenced in ways which mean their understandings of identity are abstracted to fit the agenda of transactivists. We have to ask critical questions about what is going on.

An imperative to dismantle transgender orthodoxy

Transgender ideology inducts children and families into the idea that contentment will elude them unless they hand their body over for social, chemical and surgical experimentation. Such interventions - absurdly in my view - promise to bring children's minds and genitals in to line with other people's expectations of the clothes they like to wear and the things they like to do. As we have seen through the wide range of discussions in this book, it cannot be guaranteed that social, chemical and / or surgical experimentation will reconcile children's feelings of gender confusion. The children and young people whose bodies are medically intervened in accordance with transgender doctrine are part of a speculative project in social and biological engineering. Such interventions turn a healthy child in to a life-long medical patient dependent on endless doctor visits, blood draws, radioactive scans and permanent reliance on medication. There is no public debate about the serious issues involved in transitioning children.

Many people are unaware that a child can be diagnosed as transgender before he or she knows the first thing about the meanings of gender or sex (4thwavenow, 2016). Few parents are prepared for their sons to start school and be proactively taught they might be girls. Most parents are not aware they might turn up for their daughter's school review to find she has been re-designated a boy without them knowing (as happened to GenderCriticalDad, this volume). There is no public recognition that children and adolescents are unlikely to fully comprehend the consequences for their future lives that come with hormone therapy including, but not restricted to, the risk of restricted growth, weight gain, fertility issues and mental health decline (Steensma et al, 2017). Even if children could weigh up future consequences, the long-term outcomes are not known for the health and happiness of transmen living, for example, with a prolapsed vagina and a hairy back, or the wellbeing of transwomen living with a constructed vaginal cavity as a wound that continuously tries to close, or with cancer tied to hormone use. Robust information is simply not yet available to adequately inform children and young people identifying as transgender in the pursuit of imagined gender gratification. Until such robust information is available for public scrutiny, I argue that the work of 'waiting' undertaken by some parents – going against all current guidance on transgender identification – offers a different wisdom to children and young people that supports them without reading them as 'wrong', without putting their bodies at risk and without constraining their chosen expression of gender identity:

> 'Parents who have personally observed their teens voluntarily desisting from a trans identity are the ones who have actually bought time for their kids: precious time to realize that becoming a lifelong patient haunting the offices of endocrinologists and plastic surgeons is not the only way to live a gender-defiant life
> (Overwhelmed et al, 2016).

Conclusion

I am concerned that parents have nowhere to turn for sensible and careful discussion about alternatives to social and medical intervention. I argue that the welfare and rights of children are not served by transgender doctrine which misappropriates notions of inclusion deployed by disability rights campaigners and actually undermines struggles for inclusive society. Transgenderism erodes basic principles of social justice such as health and well-being, freedom of self-expression and self-determination, respect for individuality and an acceptance of difference in all spheres of life. On the basis of my research, and having read the preceding chapters of this book, I contend that the current rise in diagnosis of gender non-conforming children as 'transgender' is antithetical to inclusion. Transgender doctrine does not, as is asserted by transgender theorists, bridge the gap between social justice, marginalization and exclusion but is forcing a chasm between the agendas of social justice and inclusion. Transgender doctrine will not smooth the path to inclusion for children and young people who experience gender dysphoria; rather it will aggressively shore up new exclusions.

Only when we begin to wrestle with social definitions of gender lodged within our own minds that act as barriers to gender freedom can we begin to engage with the struggles of children and young people articulating intense gender confusion. Insistence on medical intervention at the site of a child's body betrays adult confusion around gender. Transgender ideology and intervention confers neither safety from harm, dignity or respect upon a child. Important questions need asking about why the site of intervention for resolving children's gender discomfort isn't located within critique, rather than endorsement, of the medical model and reflection on our own attachment to gender as binary.

My observation is that transgender activists are hijacking the concept of inclusion, smuggling in a discourse of tolerance around gender fluidity which is actually polemical and destructive of ordinary protections afforded to children and young people. There is no contradiction between my respect for adults who identify as transgender and my conviction that current theory and practice of transitioning children is harmful. I cannot help wondering that people who are in positions of such social power that they can be arbiters of medical intervention, social justice, human rights, compassion and learning seem to be complying with demands from trans activists that no one shall speak out for children on the possible harms of transitioning. All that is needed to create a 'transgender child' is for enough adults to agree a child is 'in the wrong body'. This brings to mind the famous quotation usually attributed to Edmund Burke; 'the only thing necessary for the triumph of evil is that good people do nothing'.

As someone whose life work has been, and always will be to advance the agenda for inclusion, I cannot collude in the irreversible harm of children to conform to an incoherent ideology that actually excludes them from their own bodies. Application of a social constructionist lens to thinking about children and transgenderism makes societal acceptance of gender non-conformity in children far easier and more comfortable for children. Not only will the gender freedoms of children and young people be expanded but they will be safer and healthier as well. Children and young people need not be subjected to transgender intervention if we are willing to transition our own beliefs about gender conformity in order to spare them the surgeon's knife.

References

Awakening Clinician (2016) *Awakening Clinician, UK: What do we think we are talking about?* https://youthtranscriticalprofessionals.org/2016/04/24/awakening-clinician-uk-what-do-we-think-we-are-talking-about

British Psychoanalytic Council (2015) *UK Organisations Unite Against Conversion Therapy: solidarity with like-minded organisations in the USA* https://www.bpc.org.uk/news/uk-organisations-unite-against-conversion-therapy-solidarity-minded-organisations-usa_Accessed 06 07 2017

Bressert, S. (2017) *Gender Dysphoria Symptoms.* Psych Central. https://psychcentral.com/disorders/gender-dysphoria-symptoms

GenderTrender (2011) *FTM's in their own words: How to Behave Male* https://gendertrender.wordpress.com/2011/07/20/ftms-in-their-own-words-how-to-behave-mal

GIRES (undated) *Who Are You?* http://gires.org.uk/assets/Penguin

Maynard, L. (206) *A Mum's Voyage Through Transtopia: A tale of love and desistance* http//4thwavenow.com/2016/12/17/a-mums-voyage-through-transtopia-helps-her-daughter-desist/

Oliver, M. (1989) Conductive Education: If It Wasn't So Sad It Would Be Funny. *Disability, Handicap & Society,* Volume 4 (2)

—. (2013) The Social Model of Disability: Thirty years on. *Disability & Society,* Volume 28 (7)

Overwhelmed et al, (2016) *The Adolescent Trans Trend: 10 Influences* https://4thwavenow.com/2016/07/18/the-adolescent-trans-trend-10-influences/

Steensma, T.D., Annelijn Wensing-Kruger,S., and Klink, D.T. (2017) How Should Physicians Help Gender-Transitioning Adolescents Consider Potential Iatrogenic Harms of Hormone Therapy? *AMA Journal of Ethics.* Volume 19, Number 8: 762-770

Stryker, S. and Aizura, A.Z. (Eds) (2013) *The Transgender Studies Reader 2*. New York: Taylor & Francis

Transgender Trend (2016a) *Conversion Therapy for Transgender People* https://www.TransgenderTrend.com/conversion-therapy-for-transgender-people

—. (2016b) *Why Do Teenage Girls Not Want To Become Women?* https://www.TransgenderTrend.com/why-do-teenage-girls-not-want-to-become-women

YouthTransCriticalProfessionals (2016) *The Real Thing in Trans* https://youthtranscriticalprofessionals.org/2016/05

4thwavenow (2015) *UK legislators told to inculcate preschoolers with gender dogma* https://4thwavenow.com/2015/09/23/uk-legislators-told-to-inculcate-preschoolers-with-gender-dogma

—. (2016) *Gender-affirmative therapist: Baby who hates barrettes = trans boy; questioning sterilization of 11-year olds same as denying cancer treatment* https://4thwavenow.com/2016/09/29/gender-affirmative-therapist-baby-who-hates-barrettes-trans-boy-questioning-sterilization-of-11-year-olds-same-as-denying-cancer-treatment/

—. (2017) *MtoF tells trans kids to dump moms on Mother's Day and join the "glitter-queer" family of adult trans activists* https://4thwavenow.com/2017/05/14/mtof-tells-trans-kids-to-dump-moms-on-mothers-day-and-join-the-glitter-queer-family-of-adult-trans-activists